AF556860

Therapeutic Strategies

TARGETED THERAPIES IN BREAST CANCER

Therapeutic Strategies

TARGETED THERAPIES IN BREAST CANCER

Edited by

George W. Sledge, Jr.
José Baselga

CLINICAL PUBLISHING

OXFORD

Clinical Publishing
an imprint of Atlas Medical Publishing Ltd
10 Innovation House, Parkway Court
Oxford Business Park South, Oxford OX4 2JY, UK
Tel: +44 1865 811116
Fax: +44 1865 251550
Email: info@clinicalpublishing.co.uk
Web: www.clinicalpublishing.co.uk

Distributed in USA and Canada by:
Clinical Publishing
30 Amberwood Parkway
Ashland OH 44805, USA
Tel: 800-247-6553 (toll free within US and Canada)
Fax: 419-281-6883
Email: order@bookmasters.com

Distributed in UK and Rest of World by:
Marston Book Services Ltd
PO Box 269, Abingdon
Oxon OX14 4YN, UK
Tel: +44 1235 465500
Fax: +44 1235 465555
Email: trade.orders@marston.co.uk

First published 2013

A catalogue record for this book is available from the British Library.

ISBN 13 978 1 84692 066 0
ISBN e-book 978 1 84692 624 2

Project manager: Gavin Smith
Typeset by Mizpah Publishing Services Private Limited, Chennai, India
Printed by Marston Book Services Ltd, Abingdon, Oxfordshire, UK

Cover image courtesy of Derek Power BSc, MRCP, Mercy University Hospital, Cork, Ireland. Previously published in: O'Donnell, Leahy, Marples, Protheroe, Selby (eds.), *Problem Solving in Oncology*, 2007; © Clinical Publishing

Contents

Editors

GEORGE W. SLEDGE, JR., MD, Professor, Department of Medicine; Chief, Division of Oncology, Stanford University School of Medicine, Palo Alto, California, USA

JOSÉ BASELGA, MD, PhD, Physician-in-Chief, Memorial Sloan-Kettering Cancer Center, New York City, New York, USA

Contributors

ROBERT AUDET, PhD, V M Institute of Research, Montréal, Quebec, Canada

SUNIL BADVE, MD, FRCPath, Professor, Pathology and Laboratory Medicine and Internal Medicine, Indiana University Health Pathology Laboratory, Indianapolis, Indiana, USA

ADITYA BARDIA, MD, MPH, Attending Physician, Massachusetts General Hospital Cancer Center, Boston, Massachusetts, USA

RENATA DUCHNOWSKA, MD, PhD, Military Institute of Medicine, Warsaw, Poland

YESIM GÖKMEN-POLAR, PhD, Department of Medicine, Indiana University School of Medicine, Indianapolis, Indiana, USA

BRIAN LEYLAND-JONES, MD, PhD, Edith Sanford Breast Cancer Research, Sioux Falls, South Dakota, USA

CHANGYU SHEN, PhD, Division of Biostatistics, Indiana University School of Medicine, Indianapolis, Indiana, USA

D. LAWRENCE WICKERHAM, MD, National Surgical Adjuvant Breast and Bowel Project, Pittsburgh, Pennsylvania, USA

SCOOTER WILLIS, PhD, Edith Sanford Breast Cancer Research, Sioux Falls, South Dakota, USA

Acronyms and abbreviations

17-AAG	17-allylamino-17-demethoxy-geldanamycin
4HPR	N-4-hydroxyphenyl
5-FU	fluorouracil
5′-DFUR	5′-deoxy-5-fluorouridine
ACOSOG	American College of Surgeons Oncology Group
ADC	antibody-drug conjugate
ADCC	antibody-dependent cell-mediated cytotoxicity
ADH	atypical ductal hyperplasia
AI	aromatase inhibitor
AJCC	American Joint Committee on Cancer
ALDH1	aldehyde dehydrogenase 1
ALH	atypical lobular hyperplasia
ALK	anaplastic lymphoma kinase
ALTTO	Adjuvant Lapatinib and/or Trastuzumab Treatment Optimisation
AMP	adenosine monophosphate
APHINITY	Adjuvant Pertuzumab and Herceptin IN Initial TherapY of Breast Cancer
ASCO	American Society of Clinical Oncology
ATP	adenosine triphosphate
AVADO	Avastin And Docetaxel
AVEREL	AVastin in combination with hERceptin/docetaxEL in HER2-positive metastatic breast cancer
BMD	bone mineral density
BOLERO	Breast cancer trials of OraL EveROlimus
CAP	College of American Pathologists
CES-D	Center for Epidemiologic Studies Depression Scale
CHD	coronary heart disease
CI	confidence interval
CLEOPATRA	CLinical Evaluation Of Pertuzumab And TRAstuzumab
CLSI	Clinical and Laboratory Standard Institute
CNA	copy number alterations
CNS	central nervous system
COE	Center of Excellence
CORE	Continuing Outcomes Relevant to Evista
COX	cyclooxygenase
CTL	cytotoxic T lymphocyte
DAB	3,3'-diaminobenzidine
DCIS	ductal carcinoma in situ
dCK	deoxycytidine kinase
dFdCMP	fluourodeoxycytidine monophosphate
dFdCTP	2′-2′-difluourodeoxycytidine triphosphate
DFS	disease-free survival

DHFR	dihydrolate reductase
DPYD	dihydropyrimidine dehydrogenase
DVT	deep vein thrombosis
EGFR	epidermal growth factor receptor
EMILIA	An Open-Label Study of Trastuzumab Emtansine (T-DM1) vs Capecitabine+Lapatinib in Patients With HER2-Positive Locally Advanced or Metastatic Breast Cancer
EMT	epithelial-mesenchymal transition
ER	estrogen receptor
ERK1/2	extracellular signal regulated kinase
FDA	Food and Drug Administration
FDR	false discovery rate
FdUMP	fluorodeoxyuridine monophosphate
FFPE	formalin-fixed paraffin embedded
FISH	fluorescent in situ hybridization
FUTP	fluorouridine triphosphate
GM-CSF	granulocyte macrophage colony-stimulating factor
GO	gene ontology
GSEA	gene set enrichment analysis
GST	glutathione S-transferase
GWAS	genome-wide association study
hCNT	human concentrative transporter
hENT	human equilibrative transporter
HER	human epidermal growth factor receptor
hNT	human nucleotide transporter
HOT	HRT Opposed to low-dose Tamoxifen
HR	hazard ratio
Hsp90	heat shock protein 90
IBIS	International Breast Cancer Intervention Study
IGF-1	insulin-like growth factor 1
IgG	immunoglobulin G
IHC	immunohistochemical
LCIS	lobular carcinoma in situ
LDL	low-density lipoprotein
mAb	monoclonal antibody
MARIANNE	A Study of Trastuzumab Emtansine (T-DM1) Plus Pertuzumab/ Pertuzumab Placebo Versus Trastuzumab [Herceptin] Plus a Taxane in Patients With Metastatic Breast Cancer
MEK1/2	mitogen-activated extracellular-signal regulated kinase
MINDACT	Microarray In Node-negative and 1-3 node positive Disease may Avoid ChemoTherapy
MORE	Multiple Outcomes of Raloxifene Evaluation
MOS	Medical Outcomes Study
NCI	National Cancer Institute
NCIC-CTG	National Cancer Institute of Canada Clinical Trials Group
NeoALTTO	Neoadjuvant Lapatinib and/or Trastuzumab Treatment Optimisation
NSABP	National Surgical Adjuvant Breast and Bowel Project
OR	odds ratio
OS	overall survival
PAM	prediction analysis of microarrays
pCR	pathologic complete response

PCR	polymerase chain reaction
PDGF	platelet-derived growth factor
PDK1	phosphoinositide-dependent kinase 1
PE	pulmonary embolism
PEARL	Postmenopausal Evaluation and Risk-reduction with Lasofoxifene
PEPI	preoperative endocrine prognostic index
PET	positron emission tomography
PFS	progression-free survival
PIP2	phosphatidylinositol 4,5-diphosphate
PIP3	phosphatidylinositol 3,4,5-triphosphate
pNR	pathologic no response
pPR	pathologic partial response
PR	progesterone receptor
PTEN	phosphatase and tensin homolog
QA	quality assurance
QOL	quality of life
qRT-PCR	quantitative reverse transcriptase polymerase chain reaction
RCB	residual cancer burden
ROR	risk of recurrence
RR	relative risk
RUTH	Raloxifene Use for the Heart
SAM	significance analysis of microarrays
SERM	selective estrogen receptor modulator
SF-36	Short Form Health Survey
SNP	single nucleotide polymorphism
STAR	Study of Tamoxifen and Raloxifene
TAILOR x	Trial Assigning IndividuaLized Options for Treatment (Rx)
T-DM1	trastuzumab-DM1
TEACH	Tykerb Evaluation After Chemotherapy
TIA	transient ischemic attack
TNBC	triple-negative breast cancer
TOP2A	topoisomerase II alpha
TRYPHAENA	Trastuzumab plus Pertuzumab in Neoadjuvant HER2-Positive Breast Cancer
TTP	time to progression
TYMP	thymidine phosphorylase
TYMS	thymidylate synthase
VEGF	vascular endothelial growth factor
WG-DASL	Whole Genome cDNA-mediated Annealing, Selection extension and Ligation

1

The new biology of breast cancer and its therapeutic implications

G. W. Sledge Jr.

INTRODUCTION

Breast cancer therapy has undergone a series of evolutionary (and sometimes revolutionary) steps, a process that has accelerated in the past two decades as our understanding of breast cancer biology has steadily improved. This chapter, and indeed this book, outline some of these changes and attempt to place them in the context of breast cancer biology.

It is important to recognize that breast cancer therapy, from its earliest days in the modern scientific period of medicine, has always had both a strong theoretical as well as a pragmatic and empirical basis. If one begins with the last years of the nineteenth century, two theories of breast cancer biology were already being examined for their therapeutic benefit.

First, and the dominant strand for over half a century, was the work of Halsted and colleagues, who posited that breast cancer was a disease with a logical basis of metastasis via direct extension from the breast to the regional lymph nodes to distant sites via the lymphatic system. This theoretical conception of breast cancer biology implied the necessity for complete removal of all local–regional disease, and served as the basis for both breast cancer surgery and radiation therapy as potentially curative modalities.

The second strand, and ultimately the most important one for our purposes, was the recognition by Sir George Beatson that many breast cancers, though not all, were under the control of the ovaries in premenopausal women, and that breast cancers (both in the breast and at distant sites) could regress if the ovaries were resected [1]. This deep insight was ignored and forgotten for many years, but eventually served as the basis for our modern understanding of breast cancer biology.

BREAST CANCER AS A FAMILY OF DISEASES

The modern synthesis of breast cancer biology began with the discovery of the estrogen receptor (ER) in the 1960s, and the recognition by the mid-1970s that the ER could be measured in human breast cancers and predicted therapeutic response to manipulations of the internal hormonal milieu [2]. The recognition that the ER played a key role in many breast cancers also led to the development of numerous agents targeting either the ER or its ligand, estrogen.

George W. Sledge, Jr., MD, Professor, Department of Medicine; Chief, Division of Oncology, Stanford University School of Medicine, Palo Alto, California, USA.

These agents included, famously, the selective ER modulator tamoxifen, an agent which perhaps represented the first real molecularly-targeted therapy in all of oncology, and to this day the agent that has arguably saved more lives than any other in all of oncology.

Tamoxifen was followed by numerous other agents (e.g. aromatase inhibitors, LHRH agonists, fulvestrant; and steroidal agents in the progesterone, androgen, and estrogen families), but serves as an excellent example of targeted therapy. First, measure the target (in this case, the ER, though the progesterone receptor was soon added as a measure of an intact ER pathway); then use the target to determine which patients were likely to benefit from an endocrine manipulation; and then, finally, apply agents that specifically interfere with either estrogen production or the ER itself.

Though initially limited to the treatment of metastatic breast cancer, tamoxifen and its therapeutic relatives were eventually drafted for other therapeutic purposes. These have included, first and most importantly, the treatment of micrometastatic disease in the adjuvant setting, but have also included use as chemoprevention and as neoadjuvant (preoperative) therapy. Large randomized controlled trials have repeatedly demonstrated the benefits for these agents in every setting.

In both the early and advanced stages of ER-positive breast cancer, drug resistance remains a major issue. Numerous potential causes of resistance to ER-targeted therapy have been evaluated in the laboratory, as described in this volume. Few therapeutic approaches have emerged from these analyses for clinical use. An exception has been the description of the molecular target of rapamycin (mTOR) as a final common nodal point for several growth factor receptors implicated in resistance to endocrine therapy. Recently this has led to the development and evaluation of the mTOR inhibitor everolimus in combination with second-line aromatase inhibitor therapy using exemestane. The combination of these two agents is superior to exemestane alone with regard to progression-free survival in metastatic ER-positive breast cancer [3].

By the 1980s several facts became evident. While ER positivity was common in breast cancer, it was not ubiquitous. Many breast cancers clearly lacked an ER, and among those that had it, not all responded to endocrine manipulation. The search therefore began for other stimulants of breast cancer growth, and for mechanisms of resistance to ER-targeted therapy. This search led to the discovery of the second great driver of breast cancer growth, the human epidermal growth factor receptor type 2, or HER2 as it is more commonly known.

HER2 over-expression, in contrast to ER positivity, was primarily a matter of amplification of the portion of the long arm of chromosome 17 that carries the *HER2* gene. The end result of this amplification was the increased expression of HER2 on the cell membrane. This trans-membrane receptor kinase, when activated via dimerization with either other HER2 molecules or with other members of the epidermal growth factor receptor family, affected numerous intracellular functions, but particularly two major signal pathways: mitogen-activated protein (MAP) kinase and phosphoinositide 3-kinase (PI3K). Inhibition of MAP kinase and PI3K resulted in cell growth arrest and apoptosis, respectively.

HER2 amplification was initially demonstrated to be associated with impaired outcome for patients with early stage breast cancer in 1987 [4]. By the mid 1990s this observation had been amply confirmed in numerous pathological studies. It only awaited the development of a therapeutic agent to exploit this for clinical intent. The first agent to be developed in this regard was the humanized monoclonal antibody trastuzumab, which binds to the external membrane domain of the HER2 molecule.

The development of trastuzumab paralleled the earlier course pioneered by ER-based therapeutics. First, measure the receptor in human breast cancers. In the case of the ER, measurement eventually fixed on immunohistochemical analysis of the nuclear receptor. HER2, in contrast, could be measured either at the protein level (by immunohistochemical staining of the cell surface membrane receptor), or at the DNA level via fluorescence *in situ* hybridization (know as FISH; commonly expressed as a ratio of *HER2* to chromosome 17).

Measurement of HER2 was, and remains, a controversial subject, though standardization of HER2 testing (via the American Society of Clinical Oncology/College of American Pathologists guidelines) has improved HER2 testing significantly in recent years.

Next, following measurement of the HER2 molecule, treat the patients with an agent specific to HER2. Though trastuzumab was the initial HER2-targeting therapy, and remains the most commonly used agent for HER2 [5], other agents have followed. These have included, though certainly are not limited to, the small molecule receptor kinase inhibitor lapatinib [6], the monoclonal antibody pertuzumab (which interferes with HER2 dimerization with other members of the HER family) [7], and the trastuzumab-maytansanoid conjugate T-DM1 (essentially using trastuzumab to deliver a cytotoxic agent to HER2-positive breast cancer) [8].

HER2-based therapeutics followed the path trod by ER-based therapeutics in another important way. After initial positive trial results in the metastatic disease setting, trastuzumab was rapidly moved to the micrometastatic disease setting in a set of parallel trials [9, 10]. All of these trials were strikingly positive, with results suggesting that appropriate therapeutic targeting in a well-defined breast cancer subset could offer important advantages for the conduct of clinical trials. In contrast to older trials in unselected patient populations, HER2 adjuvant trials were virtually all over-powered from a statistical standpoint; such was the potency of the intervention.

The first generation of adjuvant trials also explored important questions regarding HER2 therapeutics. What represents the appropriate duration of therapy? What represents the optimal chemotherapeutic combination? Should that combination include an anthracycline, perhaps improving efficacy, but definitely increasing cardiac toxicity and with long-term effects yet to be well defined? These questions remain problematic and controversial, though answers to some important questions (particularly duration of therapy) are now beginning to emerge.

The development of later generations of HER2-targeted drugs, and in parallel an improved understanding of HER2 biology, has opened up both new questions and novel therapeutic opportunities. Partial or complete resistance to trastuzumab is ultimately quite common in metastatic disease, and remains an important cause of death in the micrometastatic disease setting. Should we, in addition to targeting the extracellular membrane receptor, also block either the downstream receptor kinase domain, or alternatively interfere with dimerization with other members of the HER family? Preclinical studies have suggested that both approaches might help prevent the development of resistance to trastuzumab.

This increased understanding of resistance mechanisms, as well as the availability of new agents developed in the metastatic disease setting, has led to the creation of several adjuvant trials examining the benefits of combined blockade of the HER2 pathway. Both health care professionals and their patients anxiously await the results of these trials. Are we close to closing the door on HER2-positive disease as a major cause of breast cancer mortality? If so, therapeutic targeting of HER2 will have been a signal success in the human cancer story.

A curious thing happened in the past decade. Oncologists had long been aware of the fact that many human breast cancers lacked either estrogen-driven or HER2-driven cancer biology. Yet these cancers had never been explored to any significant extent, either as a biological mechanism or specific clinical subset worthy of focused investigation. The demonstration of HER2- and ER-driven breast cancers (and, indeed, by cancers driven by both) ultimately focused the attention of cancer researchers on patients incapable of benefiting from either therapeutic approach.

In recent years these cancers have been colloquially known as 'triple negative breast cancer' (interestingly, the term did not enter the medical literature until the past decade). Such cancers had several defining characteristics. They tended to be poorly differentiated tumors characterized by high proliferative capacity and an increased likelihood of early distant metastasis. Though these were often sensitive to adjuvant systemic chemotherapy (the only therapy available in routine practice), in the overt metastatic setting chemotherapy proved a progressively weaker asset, with rapidly diminishing returns and the emergence of multi-drug resistance.

Most troubling, both to patients and physicians, is the fact that chemotherapeutic agents are notoriously unselective in their effects. We cannot, in simple terms, define a population that will routinely benefit from, say, paclitaxel as opposed to doxorubicin. We therefore treat patients with agents that will not work for the majority of patients in hope that some will benefit, exposing all to the very real toxic effects. In this regard, triple negative breast cancer therefore represents an area of biologic uncertainty, ethical complexity and therapeutic uncertainty.

THE GENOMIC ERA IN BREAST CANCER THERAPEUTICS

Curiously, while relatively little progress has been made regarding the targeting of specific chemotherapy agents, significant progress has occurred in predicting general chemotherapy benefit, particularly in patients with ER-positive early stage breast cancer. This progress has come about largely through the application of novel genomic technology to the breast cancer problem.

If, by the turn of the millennium, breast cancer had resolved itself into a family of diseases, characterized by distinct biologies requiring separate therapeutic approaches, what was the ultimate basis for these differences? Genomic studies using early RNA microarray technology suggested an underlying biological basis for the divisions seen in breast cancer [11]. Initial studies suggested that breast cancer could be divided into four (or perhaps five) families: Luminal A and B, basal (or basaloid), HER2, and (perhaps) normal.

In particular, Luminal A and B appeared to describe populations of ER-positive breast cancer patients with either relative lesser (Luminal A) or greater (Luminal B) proliferative capacity. Several multigene assays were developed during the past decade, and used to examine therapeutic benefit as well as evaluate overall prognosis. As a meta-analysis of these assays has shown, a proliferative gene cassette appears to be a common element predicting outcome.

One such assay, the 21-gene OncotypeDX assay, may serve as an exemplar for this approach. Analysis of early adjuvant chemotherapy trials in ER-positive lymph node-negative patients (NSABP B-14 and B-20) allowed one to determine whether a patient was at greater or lesser risk for early recurrence, and (perhaps more importantly) which patients appeared to derive benefit from the administration of adjuvant chemotherapy [12, 13]. As the hazard ratio for chemotherapy benefit in a high recurrence score subset was equivalent or superior to the hazard ratio for benefit seen with trastuzumab in HER2-positive breast cancer, adjuvant chemotherapy suddenly became a form of targeted therapy for such patients. This has fundamentally changed our approach to treatment in ER-positive, lymph node-negative patients, a population where the previous standard of care had been the application of chemotherapy to all patients with primary cancers >1 cm. The best way to avoid unnecessary toxicity is to omit treatment for patients who will not benefit from therapy.

Similar genomic analyses have been applied to earlier stage breast cancer. Evaluation of ECOG E5194 ductal carcinoma *in situ* tumor samples has suggested that a gene signature that emphasizes a proliferation cassette of genes predicts patients at increased risk for local recurrence following lumpectomy alone, and may describe a population of patients who can be spared post-lumpectomy radiation.

Subsequent genomic studies have used so-called 'deep sequencing' to evaluate early stage breast cancer, with the recent production of a veritable cornucopia of data, as organizations such as The Cancer Genome Atlas consortium (TCGA) and the International Cancer Genome Consortium (ICGC) have evaluated literally thousands of breast cancers. In general, these studies have confirmed the broad outlines of previous first-generation mRNA-based studies, suggesting that the so-called 'intrinsic subtypes' had a real genetic basis. But they have also suggested a deeper level of complexity that was previously only suspected.

The hope underlying deep sequencing of the cancer genome was that, similar to *BCR-ABL* in chronic myelogenous leukemia, we might be able to identify actionable driver mutations. But while several novel driver mutations have been identified by recent studies (in genes such as *AKT2, ARID1B, CASP8, CDKN1B, MAP3K1, MAP3K13, NCOR1, SMARCD1* and *TBX3*), there is no dominant driver mutation that suggests a panacea for any breast cancer subtype. Instead, it is the sheer complexity of the mutational landscape that impresses: looking at 100 cancers, one such study found driver mutations in at least 40 cancer genes and 73 different combinations of mutated cancer genes. The authors went on to note that, "Thus, most breast cancers differed from all others." [14] There were numerous differences seen amongst these 100, with 28 cases having only a single identifiable driver, but some having as many as six. Modern medicine has never intentionally targeted six different mutational drivers at one time, suggesting the difficulty of the task ahead of us.

Serena Nik-Zainal of the International Cancer Genome Consortium recently published a paper entitled *The Life History of 21 Breast Cancers*, analyzing breast cancers as living, evolving, dynamic cell populations [15]. Their modeling suggests that each individual breast cancer has a "most recent common ancestor" (a term derived from evolutionary biology) that occurred early in the molecular history of the cancer, and that most of the cancer's history is spent "driving subclonal diversification and evolution among the nascent cancer cells". These subclones persist until the evolutionary pressures occurring in a cancer result in one subclone eventually becoming dominant. Many mutations may occur before this dominant subclone emerges: in one case described by Nik-Zainal *et al*, the dominant subclone (65% of the cancer) had ~15,600 mutations present. The paper concludes "... we glimpse a model of long-lived, but sparse, lineages of cells passively accumulating mutations until provoked into a major quest for tumor dominance. It is only when this subclone has grown sufficiently populous that the tumor mass becomes clinically detectable."

Unsurprisingly, genomic alterations may affect therapeutic outcome. Ellis and colleagues obtained breast cancer tissue from patients treated with preoperative letrozole, then performing deep genomic sequencing to discern patterns of response and resistance. [16] Their first finding was that resistance is a *quantitative* as well as a *qualitative* problem: resistant tumors had twice as many mutations as sensitive tumors. The second finding is a daunting one: many separate mutational events were associated with resistance to hormonal therapy.

The availability of genomic analysis is rapidly increasing, a function of the plummeting cost of DNA sequencing. We are only a few years away from a time when every patient's cancer will provide informative data on the specific genetic basis for that cancer's biology. How such genomic analyses will be applied in real-life clinical scenarios represents a major challenge for the next decade.

PHARMACOGENOMICS: THE HOST GENOME AND THERAPEUTIC RESPONSE

The host genome represents a novel area of exploration for cancer researchers. Clinicians have known for decades that human variability affects patient response to systemic therapy, but it has only been in recent years that our improving technology has allowed us to study the effects of host genomic variability on therapeutic outcome (pharmacogenomics) through examination of single nucleotide polymorphisms (SNPs). In theory, genomic variability could affect both toxicity due to inborn differences in drug metabolism, and efficacy (to the extent that host variability affects drug concentration).

Numerous such SNP analyses have been performed in recent years. Perhaps the greatest effort to date has been expended on the effect of host variability in the cytochrome p450 enzyme, cyp2D6, on tamoxifen metabolism. While this literature has been both confusing and contentious, current data do not suggest that cyp2D6 SNP measurements are ready for routine clinical use.

As with tumor genomics, measurements of the host genome have become significantly less expensive in recent years, leading to an explosion of clinical study analyses. Many of these are ongoing, and evaluating large clinical trials, so it is reasonable to expect that progress will be rapid in coming years.

However, the story revealed by host genomics is likely to be a complicated one, with few simple answers. The 1000 Genomes Project recently examined the genomes of 1092 people from 14 populations around the globe. [17] The investigators discovered some 38 million SNPs (twice the previous known number), many of them quite rare, as well as 1.4 million short insertions and deletions, and some 14,000 larger deletions and rearrangements. The average person carries 76–190 rare deleterious variants expected to affect protein function, plus 20 more loss of function and disease-associated SNPs. Both the high frequency of rare variants, and the large number of deleterious variants seen, suggest that host variability will be a difficult and complicated story, and one that will require extensive study if we are to avoid misapplication of this promising technology.

ANTIANGIOGENIC THERAPY: A BLIND ALLEY?

One area that seemed immensely promising only a few years ago now seems much less so. We have know for many years that angiogenesis, or new blood vessel formation, is one of the central hallmarks of cancer biology, and that measures of angiogenesis were associated with impaired outcome. A large body of research evaluated the biology of angiogenesis, and implicated the vascular endothelial growth factor receptors (VEGFR) and their ligands as principle players in tumor angiogenesis [18].

These discoveries led, in the late 1990s, to the development of numerous agents targeting the VEGF/VEGFR complex. The first agent to see widespread experimental and clinical use was the humanized monoclonal antibody, bevacizumab. After an initial phase II experience suggested therapeutic activity, a large phase III trial was performed in front-line metastatic breast cancer combining bevacizumab and paclitaxel. The E2100 trial demonstrated a striking doubling in median progression-free survival for patients with metastatic breast cancer, and formed the basis for the subsequent approval of bevacizumab by regulatory agencies [19].

The story of anti-VEGF therapy in breast cancer, regrettably, did not end there. The E2100 study, while it demonstrated an improvement in progression-free survival, was not associated with an improvement in overall survival. Subsequent phase III trials with bevacizumab, while positive for progression-free survival, were less impressive than E2100 for this endpoint, and like E2100 failed to demonstrate an overall survival advantage. Taking these results and the known toxicities of bevacizumab into account, the Food and Drug Administration removed bevacizumab's breast cancer indication.

Adjuvant trials of bevacizumab are continuing, and may still reveal a role for this agent in breast cancer. Nevertheless, what has become clear in studies of bevacizumab and other anti-VEGF therapies in breast cancer is that they are not targeted therapies in any meaningful sense: we are currently unable to demonstrate a specific population of patients who benefit from this approach, despite the widespread appreciation that some patients benefit. Turning anti-VEGF therapy into targeted therapy remains an important part of the scientific agenda in breast cancer.

CONCLUSION: OUR PROMISING FUTURE

This volume represents an early, rather than a final, examination of targeted therapy in breast cancer. Early, because it is clear that our understanding of breast cancer biology is in a state of rapid evolution. We do not yet understand the proper application of either host or tumor genomics, as described above.

Similarly, other technologies are likely to alter our approach to the breast cancer patient in coming years. Combinatorial chemistry continues to produce a profusion of new agents for application in the clinic, their use to be described by our understanding of individual patient tumor and host biology. The related technologies of epigenomics and proteomics have barely been evaluated in breast cancer, and virtually never in the ultimate laboratory of large clinical trial sets. Finally, molecular imaging of breast cancer, a promising approach with obvious potential application for targeted therapy, is barely in its infancy.

What is clear is that the next few years will be an exciting period in the history of breast cancer biology, and that this new biology will have numerous therapeutic applications. This can only benefit our patients.

REFERENCES

1. Beatson G. On the treatment of inoperable cases of carcinoma of the mamma. *Lancet* 1896; 2:104–107.
2. Jenson E. On the mechanism of estrogen action. *Perspectives in Biology and Medicine* 1962; 6:47–59.
3. Baselga J, Campone M, Piccart M *et al.* Everolimus in postmenopausal hormone-receptor-positive advanced breast cancer. *N Engl J Med* 2012; 366:520–529.
4. Slamon D, Clark GM, Wong SG, Levin WJ, Ullrich A, McGuire WL. Human breast cancer: correlation of relapse and survival with amplification of the HER-2/neu oncogene. *Science* 1987; 235:177–182.
5. Slamon D, Leyland-Jones B, Shak S *et al.* Use of chemotherapy plus a monoclonal antibody against HER2 for metastatic breast cancer that overexpresses HER2. *N Engl J Med* 2011; 344:783–792.
6. Geyer C, Forster J, Lindquis TD *et al.* Lapatinib plus capecitabine for HER2-positive advanced breast cancer. *N Engl J Med* 2006; 355:2733–2744.
7. Baselga J, Cortés J, Kim S *et al.* Pertuzumab plus trastuzumab plus docetaxel for metastatic breast cancer. *N Engl J Med* 2012; 366:109–119.
8. Blackwell K, Miles D, Gianni L *et al.* Primary results from EMILIA, a phase III study of trastuzumab emtansine (T-DM1) versus capecitabine (X) and lapatinib (L) in HER2-positive metastatic breast cancer (MBC) previously treated with trastuzumab (T) and a taxane. *J Clin Oncol* 2012; 30:LBA1.
9. Piccart-Gebhart MJ, Procter M, Leyland-Jones B *et al*; Herceptin Adjuvant (HERA) Trial Study Team. Trastuzumab after adjuvant chemotherapy in HER2 positive breast cancer. *N Engl J Med* 2005; 353:1659–1672.
10. Romond E, Perez E, Bryant J *et al.* Trastuzumab plus adjuvant chemotherapy for operable HER2-positive breast cancer. *N Engl J Med* 2005; 353:1673–1684.
11. Perou C, Sorlie T, Eisen M *et al.* Molecular portraits of human breast tumours. *Nature* 2000; 406:747–752.
12. Paik S, Shak S, Tang G *et al.* A multigene assay to predict recurrence of tamoxifen-treated, node-negative breast cancer. *N Engl J Med* 2004; 351:2817–2826.
13. Paik S, Tang G, Shak S *et al.* Gene expression and benefit of chemotherapy in women with node-negative,estrogen receptor-positive breast cancer. *J Clin Oncol* 2006; 24: 3726–3734.
14. Stephens P, Tarpey P, Davies H *et al.* The landscape of cancer genes and mutational processes in breast cancer. *Nature* 2012; 486:400–406.
15. Nik-Zainal S, Van Loo P, Wedge D *et al.* The life history of 21 breast cancers. *Cell* 2012; 149:994–1007.
16. Ellis MJ, Ding L, Shen D *et al.* Whole-genome analysis informs breast cancer response to aromatase inhibition. *Nature* 2012; 486:353–360.
17. The 1000 Genomes Project Consortium. An integrated map of genetic variation from 1,092 human genomes. *Nature* 2012; 491:56–65.
18. Sledge G, Miller K. Angiogenesis and antiangiogenic therapy. *Curr Probl Cancer* 2002; 26:1–60.
19. Miller K, Wang M, Gralow J *et al.* Paclitaxel plus bevacizumab versus paclitaxel alone for metastatic breast cancer. *N Engl J Med* 2007; 357:2666–2676.

2

Biomarkers for targeted therapy in breast cancer: the role of the pathologist

S. Badve, Y. Gökmen-Polar

INTRODUCTION

Breast cancer is a heterogeneous disease associated with differences in morphology, biology, and response to therapy. In order to characterize this heterogeneity, it is necessary to assess molecular markers that identify subclasses or stage of disease. The term biomarkers is used to define *'a characteristic that is objectively measured and evaluated as an indicator of normal biological processes, pathogenic processes, or pharmacologic responses to therapeutic intervention'* [1]. In patients with breast cancer, biomarkers are used in clinical practice in a number of situations, the most common being predictive or prognostic markers and rarely pharmacogenomic processes. Pharmacokinetic and pharmacodynamic markers, although common in the research setting, are seldom used in clinical practice (Table 2.1). The biomarkers may be assessed in tissues or body fluids, such as blood (including plasma, serum), urine, or cerebrospinal fluid, and may be DNA, RNA, proteins, or carbohydrates. Depending on which marker is being studied, there may be different conditions required for collecting and handling the specimens.

BODY FLUID-BASED BIOMARKERS

Body fluid-based markers are obtained by minimal or non-invasive interventions and thus can be assessed serially or at multiple time points. In addition, the samples obtained can be quickly divided in to aliquots and stored or processed differently. The commonest examples of these are blood-derived assays, where the blood can be assessed as a whole sample or split into components such as plasma and serum. Depending on the assay, the samples can be collected under different conditions and with different preservatives. For example, blood might be allowed to clot (for collection of serum) or anticoagulate (for collection of plasma). As cellular components within the blood continue to degenerate, it is important to separate the components as quickly as possible to prevent contamination of the results and improve stability of the assay. Standard operative procedures for all aspects (preanalytical, analytical, and interpretational) of the assay can be devised and are relatively easy to follow.

Sunil Badve, MD, FRCPath, Professor, Pathology and Laboratory Medicine and Internal Medicine, Indiana University Health Pathology Laboratory, Indianapolis, Indiana, USA.

Yesim Gökmen-Polar, PhD, Department of Medicine, Indiana University School of Medicine, Indianapolis, Indiana, USA.

Table 2.1 Types of assay in clinical trials

	Biomarkers	*Examples*
Research use	Pharmacokinetic	Determination of the fate of drug
	Pharmacodynamic	Mechanisms of drug absorption; distribution of an administered drug
Clinical practice	Pharmacogenomic	CYD2D6 SNPs and tamoxifen; SULT1A1 and tamoxifen
	Prognostic	ER/PR; Ki67
	Predictive	ER/PR; HER2
	Integral	HER2 in clinical trial of Herceptin; Onco*type* DX for TAILORx
	Integrated	PTEN in clinical trial of Herceptin; Ki67 for TAILORx

PREANALYTICAL FACTORS

Preanalytical factors include all aspects of the assay process prior to the conduct of the assay itself. These include collection, preprocessing, and processing of the sample, including storage until the time of conduction of the assay.

Sample collection

The samples can be obtained in a standardized manner, including the time of the day and day of the week they were collected. This can enable detection of relatively minor degrees of variability which can contribute to greater sensitivity and specificity of the assay. This is important for assays for analytes that exhibit cyclical variations in their levels. The samples can also be collected in a uniform manner so that parameters that might interfere with the assay can be avoided. For example, fasting samples might be better than postprandial if lipids interfere with the assay.

Sample handling

Sample handling starts right from the time it is obtained/extracted from the subject/patient. Optimal care is required to ensure that it is not contaminated by other tissue fluids or environmental factors. Introduction of even small factors such as epithelial cells or air bubbles can significantly impact the assay. It is not uncommon for the sample to be set aside while the patient is being taken care of; this can also introduce errors. For example, blood collected might clot or hemolyze, giving rise to contamination of the plasma. The sample should be sent to the laboratory for analysis as early as possible. It should be stored appropriately during transportation.

Sample processing

Once a sample is received in the lab, it should either be processed immediately or stored in appropriate conditions. The processing might involve separating the sample into its constituents (as for a blood sample) and storing it in preparation for analysis.

ANALYTICAL FACTORS

The assay technology for body fluid-based analysis can be specific for the analyte and need not depend on what other assays are being performed on the same sample. This can permit fine tuning of the assay technology and the samples can be collected under optimal conditions.

ASSAY INTERPRETATION

The well-controlled nature of the sample collection, handling, processing, and analytical (total assay) methods enable exquisite sensitivity and specificity in the interpretation of samples collected from body fluids. Assay results can be measured with the best possible methods, giving the manufacturers a wide scope in assay design and implementation. This is in complete contrast to tissue-based assays described below.

TISSUE-BASED ASSAYS

Tissue-based assays are complicated by the fact that they are dependent on invasive procedures. These procedures can be minimally invasive as in fine needle biopsy of the breast, somewhat invasive as in core biopsy, or invasive as in excision specimens of tumors/lesions. The procedures cannot be repeated, either because of the procedure involved or, more commonly, because all of the lesional tissue was removed in the first procedure. This introduces limitations that affect all aspects of the assay process, as will be apparent from the discussion below. The methodologies that have been developed have been in use for decades and are not easy to change. This is in part due to tissue limitations (i.e. small tumor size or possible interference by non-tumor elements) but also because the utility (prognostic or predictive) is often established in a retrospective manner. Prospective clinical trials, although performed for drugs, have never been performed for biomarkers. Suffice to say, the analyte needs to be robust and stable over relatively long periods of time to enable tissue-based analyses. In addition, the analyte needs to be detectable in archival paraffin-embedded tissues if the assay is to have any hope of widespread clinical applicability.

PREANALYTIC VARIABLES

Sample collection

Tissue samples are mostly collected by employing invasive techniques. Depending on the procedure involved, procurement of the specimen may take from seconds to hours. Vacuum-assisted core biopsies are usually collected under close to ideal circumstances and permit for fixation within seconds. They are therefore most often used in clinical practice for assessment of biomarkers. Excision biopsy and mastectomy procedures can last for hours. More importantly, the main feeder vessel supplying the tumor area may be ligated or cauterized long before the entire specimen is taken out. This can result in significantly prolonged 'warm ischemia'. It is very difficult to control this warm ischemia time, but what can be controlled is the time interval between removal of the specimen and its placement in formalin. Although some studies have suggested that a delay to specimen fixation of less than 12 hours at room temperature or 4°C does not significantly alter immunostaining [2–4], this is not acceptable. The American Society of Clinical Oncology–College of American Pathologists (ASCO–CAP) guidelines recommend that this interval should be less than 1 hour [5].

Sample handling

The goal of the clinical staff should be to deliver the specimen to the pathology lab in as pristine condition as possible. If delivery of fresh specimen is not possible, it is recommended that the specimen should be delivered in 'neutral buffered formalin'. Buffering of the formalin with a phosphate buffer to pH 5 to 7 is optimal for immunohistochemistry [3, 5–8]. It is generally recommended that the ratio of tissue to formalin should be in the range of 1:10 [5, 7]. If the specimen cannot be delivered quickly, it should be sliced into thin slices

(~5 mm) and then placed in formalin to permit infiltration and fixation of the tumor. Slicing of the specimen by surgeons can lead to difficulties in assessment of the margin status. Coordination with the pathologist with regards to inking of the specimen by the surgical team or slicing the specimen is required to circumvent these difficulties.

Once the specimen is received in the lab, it should be inked and sliced as soon as possible and thin slices should be placed in formalin. Placement of gauze or paper between the slices can aid the process of fixation. Underfixation as well as overfixation can affect the quality of marker analysis. National guidelines vary in different countries but a fixation time of between 6 and 72 hours is acceptable as per the ASCO–CAP guidelines [5, 8]. It has been suggested in some studies that fixation can be hastened by microwaving the tissue or by the use of ultrasound [9–14]. The recommendations of the Clinical and Laboratory Standard Institute (CLSI) [7] describe the characteristics of specimens that might be suitable for microwave fixation. These include:

1. Tissues less than 5 mm in thickness.
2. Tissues immersed in formalin for less than 4 hours.
3. Tissues microwaved in formalin for 5 minutes or less in 100 ml of formalin.

These methods are still experimental in nature and have not been approved for clinical use.

Several fixatives that are alternative to formalin have been proposed and are in use. This is particularly true in France, where formalin is classified as a carcinogen. The principal alternatives are alcohol-based. In general, these are not recommended for use as they might interfere with testing for estrogen receptor/progesterone receptor (ER/PR) and human epidermal growth factor receptor (HER2). In the United States, the kits for HER2 are only FDA approved for formalin-fixed, paraffin-embedded tissues.

Sample processing

The main function of specimen processing is to make the tissue hard enough to cut on the microtome and obtain thin sections. It involves dehydration of the tissue using serial exposure to varying concentrations of methanol followed by xylene, which is miscible with paraffin wax. Fatty tissues such as the breast are more difficult to process and longer processing times are often needed to get optimal results. The impact of the reagents used with biomarker analysis has not been well studied [8]. However, it is undoubted that these parameters play a role. This variability is usually compensated by altering the timing of exposure to enzymes (such as proteases in fluorescent *in situ* hybridization (FISH) and immunohistochemistry (IHC) analysis) and by altering the time of antigen retrieval.

A number of alternative processing methods have been tested. These include the use of the different alcohols, acetone, or alternative solutions to dehydrate the tissues. The use of these alternatives can provide for faster processing times. Some commercially available techniques and products can process the tissue in a couple of hours. Preliminary results with some of the products are promising in terms of concordance with routine processing. However, large-scale testing has not been done. In addition, most of these studies do not have a therapeutic endpoint.

Although the type of paraffin wax (polymer, non-polymer, and microcrystalline) used does not affect immunostaining [3], its melting temperature has been shown to have an impact on the extent and intensity of the immunostaining [2]. Some guidelines recommend the use of wax with a melting point of 55–58°C.

Variables related to section cutting have not been examined in detail. Adhesives that improve the adhesion of the sections to the glass slide have been examined in some detail. These chemicals do not seem to impact the quality of staining [8]. Drying of the slides at room temperature for 24 hours or at least 1 hour at 50–60°C is usually recommended [7]. Variations of these conditions have been suggested to affect the quality of staining [7, 8].

Paraffin blocks can be used for routine biomarker analysis for decades and must therefore be carefully stored [15, 16]. The quality of RNA deteriorates to some extent after 15 years but can still be used [17]. Several groups have successfully analyzed mRNA from these blocks and developed clinical assays. Storage at room temperature or in a 'cool' room is recommended. Storage of slides is a major issue. Some antigens are irretrievably lost after a few weeks of storage (e.g. ER, PR, and HER2) but others can be used decades later without significant loss of antigenicity [18–21]. Methods such as freezer storage (with silica gel dehydration packs) or redipping the slides in paraffin prior to storage have been used with some success. Storage of unstained slides in a temperature-controlled environment is generally recommended.

ANALYTIC METHODS AND INTERPRETATION

Antigen retrieval

Formalin fixation and processing leads to alterations of the protein structure and masking of the epitopes. A number of methods have been applied to 'unmask' the antigen; these are collectively referred to as antigen retrieval [22, 23]. Although many of these methods look and sound primitive (steaming or boiling tissue in buffers), they work quite well in routine practice. Specialized chambers for antigen retrieval provide more consistent results than simple (kitchen) pressure cookers or steamers. Standardized reagents and kits should be used whenever possible. Protocols to measure consistency of the reagents and lot-to-lot variability need to be in place and appropriate documentation needs to be maintained. Selection of appropriate reagents should be based on published literature using that specific clone or kit; FDA approval can serve as a good guide in the decision making.

Interpretation of the stained slides requires thorough knowledge of the histology and cannot be left to inexperienced technicians; this is particularly true for *HER2* FISH analysis. In this analysis, it is critical to identify foci of invasive carcinoma and exclude foci of *in situ* disease. It is important to visualize the entire slide to identify zones of adequate staining and exclude areas with artifacts caused either by the biopsy process or by the staining process. In group practices, it is necessary to standardize reading patterns across the entire group if the assessment cannot be restricted to a limited number of practitioners. In spite of the best precautions, assessment of certain special stains such as Ki67 remains difficult. Automated analysis systems can play a useful role in training and standardization of the reading. However, many of these still depend on the assessment of a single or multiple operator-selected foci and can be prone to operator-dependent errors. Whole slide scanners and analyzers are being introduced; these may be more reliable than the currently available systems.

ROLE OF THE PATHOLOGIST

The role of the pathologist has undergone significant expansion in the era of targeted therapeutics (Figure 2.1). The pathologist determines the expression of the target in the cancer cells and thus plays a critical role in the determination of therapy. Understanding this basic concept is important not only for the pathologist but also for the clinical team. Far too often, pathologists are regarded by the clinical teams (particularly the ancillary staff) as a source of reports and are not given any intellectual credit/role in making strategic patient management decisions. The clinical team needs to realize that the biomarker analysis is an integrative process and that specimen handling is of utmost importance in obtaining opti-

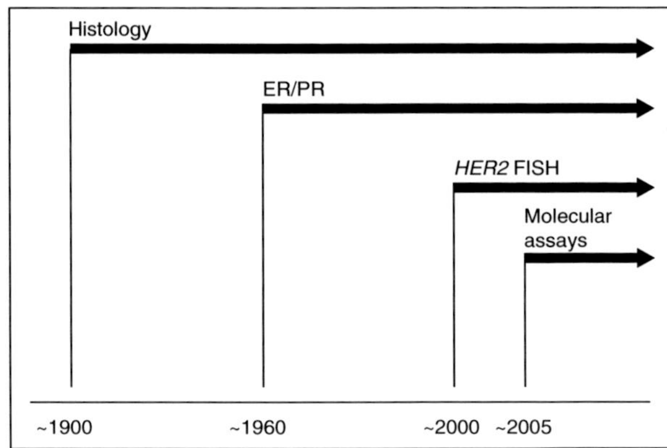

Figure 2.1 The chronological order of milestones for targeted therapy in the practice of pathology.

mal care for 'their' patient. Explaining some of these concepts to the nursing and operating room staff is often required to get their cooperation and active participation in the process.

HANDLING OF SURGICAL SPECIMENS

One of the important roles of surgical pathologists is to ensure the prompt handling of surgical specimens. As discussed above, optimal fixation and processing are critical to achieving accurate and consistent biomarker analysis. Whenever possible, an attempt should be made to collect fresh tumor and freeze it using liquid nitrogen. This is particularly important for novel biomarker discovery rather than for routine diagnostic purposes.

ASSESSMENT OF TRADITIONAL CLINICOPATHOLOGICAL PARAMETERS

Tumor size

Classic parameters, such as tumor size and tumor grade, are still integral to clinical decision making. Chemotherapy decisions are still made on the basis of tumor size, receptor expression, and nodal status. Large node-positive tumors will almost definitely be treated with chemotherapy. The management of smaller tumors is much more difficult to predict and is based on subjective decisions made with the clinician in consultation with the patient. Recent studies have shown that small (less than 1 cm) tumors with an aggressive profile (i.e. triple negative or HER2-positive phenotype) may benefit from the addition of chemotherapy [24, 25].

Histologic grade

Histologic grade is an extremely important prognostic factor [24]. The interobserver variability results show a kappa value in the range of 0.5, indicative of modest agreement [26]. This has led to clinicians questioning the value of grade as a prognostic marker. However, it should be noted that, in most studies, it still retains value as an independent prognostic marker. More importantly, the *P* values and hazard ratios for histological grade are in the same range as some of the molecular assays (e.g. Onco*type* DX; detailed later) [26, 27]. This has led to some clinicians recognizing the value of grade and use of molecular assays selectively in tumors that are grade 2 by histology. Fortunately, or unfortunately, many of these are also found to be 'intermediate' by molecular assays.

Lymph nodes

The methods for assessment of lymph nodes have significantly changed in the past decade. The adoption of a sentinel node biopsy procedure was associated with an increased number of intraoperative evaluations when making decisions regarding complete axillary dissection. The recent completion of the NSABP B32 [28] and ACOSOG Z011 [29] clinical trials has led to the questioning of the role of complete axillary dissection. This has resulted in a significant diminution of the use of intraoperative lymph node assessment, particularly for patients with disease similar to those enrolled in these clinical trials. Intraoperative assessment is still used for patients who are undergoing mastectomy and, in some cases, for patients undergoing immediate plastic reconstruction.

Margins

The assessment of margins is one of the critical components of a surgical pathology report. Proper orientation of the specimen and sampling are required to perform this task adequately. In the era of mammography, where tumor is primarily detected based on the presence of architectural abnormalities, the specimen often undergoes radiological examination prior to arrival in the laboratory. The specimen often undergoes compression ('pancaking'), resulting in artificial lengthening or shortening of the distance of the tumor from the true margin. It is necessary to note the plane of compression so that the patient does not undergo unnecessary surgery for an artificially close margin.

All other parameters

A number of prognostic indices have been used to predict behavior of breast cancers. The three most commonly used are: TNM stage (AJCC [30]), the Nottingham Prognostic Index [31], and Adjuvant Online! [32]. The TNM stage is based on the tumor size (and involvement of local structures such as chest wall and skin) and the presence or absence of nodal or systemic metastases. The Nottingham Prognostic Index combines tumor size and nodal status with tumor grade to generate a prognostic index. Adjuvant Online! takes into consideration a number of clinicopathological parameters, including patient age, tumor size, grade, ER status, and nodal involvement, to determine the risk of relapse/metastases. It also provides a rough guide to the likelihood of benefit following endocrine therapy, chemotherapy, or a combination of these. Newer versions of Adjuvant Online! that incorporate molecular assays are being developed.

ANALYSIS OF RESPONSE TO THERAPY

Post neoadjuvant chemotherapy

The pathologist is often called upon to evaluate tumor response to prior therapies. This is often difficult for the pathologist due to a lack of data regarding tumor size (prior to therapy) or, in some cases, to not acknowledging whether the patient received neoadjuvant chemotherapy. A number of methods for the assessment of clinical response to therapy have been described. Commonly used systems have been devised/described by the NSABP [33], Miller and Payne [34], Chevallier [35], Sataloff [36], and the residual cancer burden (RCB) system [37] and these are very briefly described below. The NSABP [33] system classifies patients as having pathologic complete response (pCR) if there is no evidence of residual invasive carcinoma in the tumor bed. The presence of scattered foci or single tumor cells falls under the category of pathologic partial response (pPR). The system described by Miller and Payne [34] recognizes five categories, with grade 1 indicative of minimal or no response (pNR) and grade 5 as no evidence of invasive carcinoma in the tumor bed (pCR). The presence or absence of ductal carcinoma *in situ* (DCIS) or tumor in regional lymph nodes is not considered in determination of response in the systems. The Chevallier method [35] recognizes four classes in which class 1 represents absence of both in situ disease and invasion into the breast and lymph nodes; class 2 is associated with presence of residual DCIS but no invasive tumor; and classes 3 and 4 represent partial and no response to therapy. The Sataloff method [36] separately evaluates the tumor bed and the regional lymph nodes, with subcategories (A–D) affixed to each, depending on the amount of tumor left. Subcategory A represents complete absence of tumor (pCR), while subcategory D represents no response (pNR). The RCB system [37] recognizes four categories (0–III); category RCB-0 represents no residual tumor, RCB-I represents minimal residual tumor, RCB-II represents significant residual tumor, and RCB-III is indicative of little or no response to therapy. The advantage of the RCB system is that it has been developed in the era of modern chemotherapy. The system is associated with a detailed description of the methodology and uses morphological appearances of the prior biopsy as a guide to assessing therapeutic response.

Post neoadjuvant endocrine therapy

Neoadjuvant endocrine therapy has also been used in patients with large ER-positive tumors. The preoperative endocrine prognostic index (PEPI) was developed in patients treated with aromatase inhibitors and tamoxifen prior to surgery [38]. The PEPI score was derived from the sum of the risk points weighted by the size of the hazard ratio assigned to each statistically significant factor. These factors include pathological tumor size, nodal status, Ki67 expression level, and level of ER positivity. Patients with a low score have better outcomes compared to those with higher scores.

TRADITIONAL MOLECULAR DIAGNOSTICS FOR THERAPY

The pathologist is often the only physician involved in deciding which assays are to be performed and the methodologies associated with the assays. Assay selection and performance of the test are critical functions of the pathologist. Standard US Food and Drink Administration (FDA)-approved assays should be used. However, multiple manufacturers are available for any given assay. Published data from quality assurance (QA) programs such as CAP, NORDIC QC, and UK-NEQAS should be used to guide these decisions. Participation in these (or similar) QA programs is required by the ASCO–CAP guidelines.

The choice of the assay is also somewhat dependent on the institution and payment practices. In the United States, reimbursement practices will often permit the use of premanufactured kits that include antibodies as well as detection systems. Automation is often possible but it also depends on the overall workload of the lab. Whenever possible, kits should be used, as these give optimal results. Automation goes a long way towards ensuring consistent technical results.

Assay interpretation is not always easy and is often complicated by issues such as heterogeneity. Careful attention to detail is of paramount importance. Evaluation of the entire test slide as well as the positive and negative controls is necessary. Areas with artifacts generated either due to edge effect or uneven distribution of reagents should be excluded. Similarly, assessment should be confined to areas of invasive tumor. Whenever possible, blocks that can provide for internal controls should be used for assay. There is some disagreement about whether the most differentiated tumor should be used for the analysis of ER/PR while the most undifferentiated tumor should be used for analysis of HER2. In general, the best fixed tissue should be used for the analysis. In most cases, the biopsy sample is the best preserved and markers are often performed on this sample. In cases where the biopsy sample is completely negative for the markers, additional testing may be repeated on the excision sample. In some institutions, it is standard practice to perform the testing on both biopsy and excision samples.

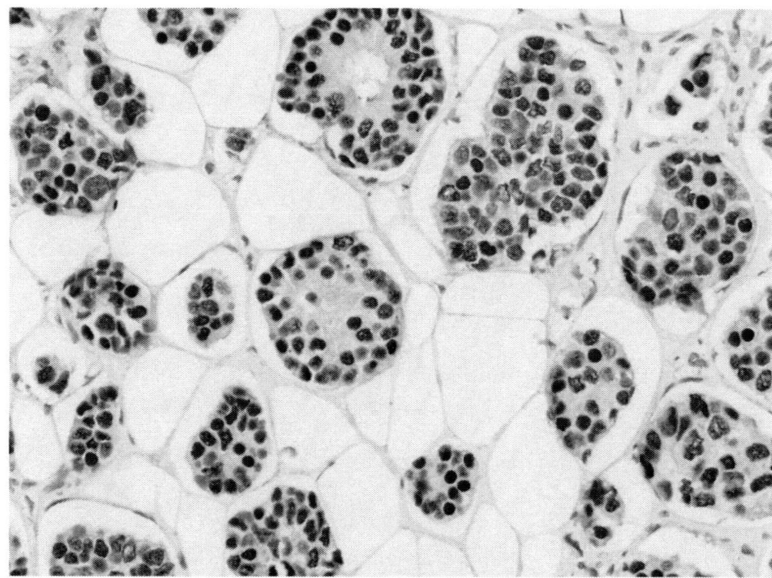

Figure 2.2 ER expression in invasive breast cancer. Note the nuclear expression of estrogen receptor in the tumor cells.

SPECIFIC ISSUES

ER/PR analysis

The analysis of ER and PR has been an integral component of the pathology report for several decades (Figure 2.2). A number of methods have been used for the analysis over this time. IHC has become the standard of practice across the world. Several FDA-approved kits are available, which include single antibodies or a combination of monoclonal antibodies (e.g. ER pharmDX™). The monoclonal antibodies (such as SP1 [39] and EP1 (Dako)) appear to be superior to the mouse monoclonal antibodies. A number of cutoff points have been used in literature ranging from 10% to any positive cells. The current ASCO–CAP guidelines recommend the use of 1% as a cutoff for positivity [5]. The recommendations also suggest reporting both the intensity and the percentage of positivity. It is recognized that patients with high ER expression are more likely to have a therapeutic response than those with low ER expression. The provision of details pertaining to ER expression should enable clinicians to make appropriate therapeutic decisions based on likelihood of response and patient-reported toxicities.

HER2 analysis

The data from the clinical trials have clearly shown the importance of HER2 in early breast cancer and in metastatic breast cancer. Analysis of this marker should be performed on each and every breast specimen. At least two methods of analysis are available; these include IHC and FISH. Both methods are associated with advantages and disadvantages; the current ASCO–CAP guidelines recommend the use of either [40] (Figure 2.3). The concordance between FISH and IHC for positive and negative cases needs to be documented and should be in the neighborhood of 95%. The guidelines recognize three broad categories for both methods: negative (IHC, 0 or 1+; FISH ratio, less than 1.8); equivocal (IHC, 2+; FISH ratio, 1.8–2.2); and positive (IHC, 3+; FISH ratio, >2.2). Cases classified as equivocal need addi-

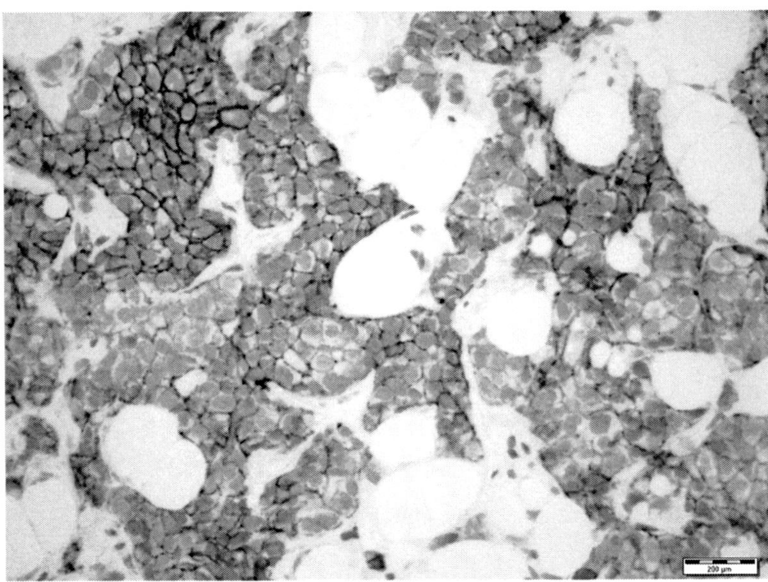

Figure 2.3 HER2 staining in breast cancer: note the membranous staining in more than 10% but less than 30% of tumors. This is considered 2+ as per the ASCO–CAP guidelines but was considered positive in clinical trials.

tional analysis to clarify the positive or negative status. It should be kept in mind that a FISH ratio of >2 was used as the eligibility criterion in the clinical trials. IHC-negative or equivocal patients with a FISH ratio >2 are still eligible for HER2 targeted therapy [41].

It would be simplistic to expect all positive cases to respond to targeted HER2 therapy. In addition, the situation is complicated by the retrospective analysis of the HER2 clinical trials, where locally positive, centrally negative cases have been documented to show a therapeutic response. Some have hypothesized that this represents a response in HER2-negative patients [42]; a randomized clinical trial is currently being conducted to clarify these issues.

Ki67 analysis

The analysis of Ki67 is complicated by the lack of good controls. A recent review has highlighted this issue in considerable detail [43]. An international working group, which includes the National Cancer Institute (NCI), has been formed to develop standard methods and practices for the performance and assessment of Ki67. Briefly, the issues not only include the choice of the reagents but also the 'regions of interest' where the analysis should be performed. Ki67 expression is often higher at the leading edge of the tumor as opposed to the central regions. This can lead to significant discordance between different assessments. In addition, there is a lack of consensus on the intensity of DAB staining required to call a cell positive.

Basal-like carcinoma markers

Molecular profiling studies in breast cancer identified a category of tumors referred to as basal-like carcinomas. There is considerable overlap between this entity and triple negative tumors. Some authors recommend further classification of triple negative tumors and those that have basal-like characteristics (for review, see Badve *et al.* [44]). Epidermal growth factor receptor (EGFR) and cytokeratin 5 are commonly used as a distinction. The cutoff points for positivity are poorly defined and tend to vary from study to study. In addition, there are no definite therapies (as of yet) for basal-like carcinomas and the utility of these stains in routine diagnostics has been questioned by some, including our group.

Metastatic lesions

There is a considerable amount of evidence that shows significant variability (~20%) between the primary tumor and the subsequent metastasis that develops in the same patient. For hormone receptors, loss of progesterone receptor is far more common than estrogen receptor. Similar high levels of discordance are reported for HER2 analysis. Studies suggest that this discordance occurs in both directions with an almost equal number of negative tumors having HER2 positivity in the metastatic sites and vice versa [45, 46].

MULTIGENE EXPRESSION PROFILE-BASED ASSAYS

Intrinsic subtypes and PAM50

Gene expression studies have shown that breast cancers can be classified into a number of molecular subtypes, some of which may have prognostic relevance. The initial studies were based on microarrays and used 'centroids' to define categories [47, 48]. This method is inherently unstable as addition of another sample to the study set leads to a shift of the centroid [49]. The assay has been recently converted into Nanostring®-based analysis of 50 genes (PAM50 assay) [50]. The output of the assay 'ROR' (risk of recurrence) takes into account tumor size in addition to the expression of these 50 genes. A recent study [51] showed superior performance of this assay as compared to Onco*type* DX assay (see below) in predicting the recurrence of ER-positive tumors treated with endocrine therapy.

Mammaprint

Researchers at the Netherland Cancer Institute, in a microarray-based analysis, found that >5000 genes were differentially expressed between good prognosis tumors and bad prognosis tumors [52, 53]. Expression of a set of 70 genes could reliably distinguish the two groups and constitutes the Mammaprint assay. However, the assay required frozen tissues and had limited market penetration. More recently, the assay has been adapted for quantitative reverse transcriptase polymerase chain reaction (qRT-PCR) and is now commercially available. The utility of the assay is being studied in the MINDACT clinical trial [54].

Oncotype DX

The investigators at the NSABP and Genomic Health Inc. used an alternative approach in which they studied the expression of a limited number of genes (~185) in archival paraffin blocks from two clinical trials (NSABP B-14 and B-20). These identified a set of 16 genes plus controls (total 21 genes), which were not only associated with prognosis but also with response to therapy [26, 27]. Patients with low recurrence scores derive the most benefit from endocrine therapy but little or no benefit from chemotherapy. Similarly, patients with high scores do not significantly benefit from endocrine therapy, but do obtain huge benefit from chemotherapy (28% absolute benefit). The utility of the assay is being studied in the TAILORx clinical trial [55, 56].

NOVEL TECHNOLOGIES AND THE EMERGING ROLE OF THE PATHOLOGIST IN THE GENOMIC ERA

Advances in gene expression profiling technologies have dramatically improved our understanding of the genomic and transcriptomic landscape of breast cancer. Most importantly, they have not only revealed the genetic diversity and complexity of breast cancer at the intertumor and intratumor levels, but have also contributed to the prognostic/predictive utility of the identified gene sets [57–60]. A recent study using gene expression and copy number variation analyses identified ten subtypes of breast cancer including basal-like cancers [61]. Another study defined six subtypes of triple negative breast cancers, a category that shows significant overlap with basal-like cancers [62]. Next generation sequencing (also called deep sequencing) studies have identified a number of mutations, mostly with a low incidence (<5%). However, some mutations (detailed below) are relatively common and are being targeted for therapeutics. This indicates that, although the incorporation of these data into clinical decisions might be a slow process, it is changing thought processes and could impact practice at least in research settings (and clinical trials) in the near future.

ASSESSMENT OF BIOMARKERS DRIVEN BY GENOMIC ALTERATIONS

Genomic technologies have not only revealed the molecular basis of breast cancer that may change clinical outcome, but have also helped to identify gene alterations that predict response to therapy. In particular, recent studies have focused on the identification of somatic mutations and copy number alterations (CNAs) in intrinsic breast cancer subtypes. Curtis *et al* [61] analyzed 2000 breast cancers, subsequently categorizing breast cancer into ten distinct subtypes containing 45 regions of sequence amplification or deletion that may control the regulation of genes important in breast cancer pathology. A number of studies in both ER-positive and triple-negative breast cancers (TNBC) have identified a few highly recurrent driver mutations as well as many low frequency mutations considered as passenger mutations [57–60]. Specifically, TNBCs showed a diverse spectrum of mutational events from one tumor to another. *TP53, PIK3CA,* and *PTEN* were among the few highly recurrent mutations involved in the early tumorigenesis. Significantly, driver mutations have also been identified in luminal breast cancers, including *PIK3CA, TP53, GATA3, CDH1,* and *MAP3K1*.

THERAPEUTIC TARGETING OF BIOMARKERS DRIVEN BY GENOMIC ALTERATIONS

The identification of driver-genetic mutations has improved the path to the development of targeted therapies that are oriented to these mutations and their pathways. Preclinical studies have reported that PIK3CA mutations, responsible for activation of the PI3K/AKT/mTOR pathway, determine the sensitivity of breast cancer cells to PI3K and mTOR inhibitors [63, 64]. Recently, other studies have emphasized *PIK3CA* and *PTEN* mutations in breast cancer subtypes including TNBCs [62, 64]. TNBC cell lines harboring mutations of PI3K/AKT signaling (*PIK3CA* mutations or *PTEN* deficiency) were highly sensitive to the dual PI3K/mTOR inhibitor, NVP-BEZ235 [62]. A prospective clinical trial sequenced *PIK3CA* in tumors from patients with advanced breast cancer and gynecologic cancers [65]. Patients with *PIK3CA* mutations treated with PI3K/AKT/mTOR inhibitors demonstrated a higher response rate (30%) than patients without mutations (10%). Another study using high-throughput RNA interference/siRNA knockdown approach for 714 human kinases identified two distinct groups, one enriched for *PTEN* mutations (group 1) and another for *PIK3CA* mutations (group 2) [66]. *PTEN*-deficient breast cancer cells require several mitotic checkpoint kinases, including the *TTK* protein kinase gene (also known as MPS1). Currently, TTK inhibitors are being developed for cancers that have a high level of chromosome instability.

The anaplastic lymphoma kinase (*ALK*) gene has been shown to be amplified in inflammatory breast cancer and small-molecule ALK inhibitors are effective in mouse xenograft models [67]. Patients with inflammatory breast cancer are now being screened for *ALK* genetic abnormalities and may be enroled in a phase 1, dose-escalation clinical trial of a small-molecule ALK/CMET inhibitor, if they contain the *ALK* amplification.

FUTURE DIRECTIONS

REDEFINING THE GROWING NEED FOR THE PATHOLOGIST IN THE ERA OF PERSONALIZED THERAPIES; THE NEW RESPONSIBILITIES OF THE PATHOLOGIST

The gene discoveries and mutation analysis data highlight new responsibilities and challenges for the pathologist. Given the fact that many of these mutations are rare, screening of a large number of tumors is necessary in order to identify the presence of therapeutically relevant mutations. However, this is not a straightforward task, as response rates, even in patients with documented mutations, can be low; 30% for patients with *PIK3CA* [65]. This may be due to the complexity of the pathways, intratumoral heterogeneity, and/or other driver mutations or alterations. In addition, experience in leukemia and gastrointestinal stromal tumors has shown that tumors can develop secondary 'adaptive' mutations that can circumvent targeted therapies. This reality emphasizes the need for tumor genetic testing not only for patient selection but also for continuous monitoring during treatment.

GENE DISCOVERY IN THE PATHOLOGY LAB

Going forward, it will be necessary to perform mutational and transcriptomic/genomic screening of tumors for selection and monitoring of targeted therapies. Pathology labs will have to perform these complex assays on a routine basis. High dependence on robotics, automated specimen handling, and automated specimen tracking will greatly simplify the management and tracking of specimens within the laboratory. However, the interpretation of these assays is unlikely to be easy and a new breed of laboratory doctors trained in these aspects of data analysis and reporting will be necessary. These 'omics' data will need to be incorporated with the traditional evaluation to obtain a comprehensive picture of the tumor. The PAM50-ROR Score and Onco*type* DX RSPC are early prototypes of this form of data reporting [50, 68]. It is not impossible to envision the pathology lab being a hub of services – including diagnostic molecular pathology, diagnostic genomics, transcriptomics, proteomics, and pharmacogenomics – in addition to the traditional histological diagnostic service. In summary, the pathologist will need to take a leadership role in bridging the disciplines and synergizing the multidisciplinary approach to cancer treatment in the era of personalized therapy. If the pathology labs and pathologists fail to meet these challenges, there is a real danger they will be bypassed in the decision-making process by the development of a new field of molecular oncology.

REFERENCES

1. Biomarkers Definitions Working Group. Biomarkers and surrogate endpoints: preferred definitions and conceptual framework. *Clin Pharmacol Ther* 2001; 69:89–95.
2. Pollard K, Lunny D, Holgate CS *et al.* Fixation, processing, and immunochemical reagent effects on preservation of T-lymphocyte surface membrane antigens in paraffin-embedded tissue. *J Histochem Cytochem* 1987; 35:1329–1338.
3. Williams JH, Mepham BL, Wright DH. Tissue preparation for immunocytochemistry. *J Clin Pathol* 1997; 50:422–428.
4. Khoury T, Sait S, Hwang H *et al.* Delay to formalin fixation effect on breast biomarkers. *Mod Pathol* 2009; 22:1457–1467.
5. Hammond ME, Hayes DF, Dowsett M *et al.* American Society of Clinical Oncology/College Of American Pathologists guideline recommendations for immunohistochemical testing of estrogen and progesterone receptors in breast cancer. *J Clin Oncol* 2010; 28:2784–2795.
6. von Wasielewski R, Mengel M, Wiese B *et al.* Tissue array technology for testing interlaboratory and interobserver reproducibility of immunohistochemical estrogen receptor analysis in a large multicenter trial. *Am J Clin Pathol* 2002; 118:675–682.

7. Lightfoote MM, Ball DJ, Hannon WH *et al.* Quality Assurance for Design Control and Implementation of Immunohistochemistry assays; Approved guideline. 2nd edition ed. Wayne PA. USA: Clinical and Laboratory Standards Institute; 2010.
8. Engel KB, Moore HM. Effects of preanalytical variables on the detection of proteins by immunohistochemistry in formalin-fixed, paraffin-embedded tissue. *Arch Pathol Lab Med* 2011; 135:537–543.
9. Chu WS, Liang Q, Tang Y *et al.* Ultrasound-accelerated tissue fixation/processing achieves superior morphology and macromolecule integrity with storage stability. *J Histochem Cytochem* 2006; 54:503–513.
10. Chu WS, Furusato B, Wong K *et al.* Ultrasound-accelerated formalin fixation of tissue improves morphology, antigen and mRNA preservation. *Mod Pathol* 2005; 18:850–863.
11. Azumi N, Joyce J, Battifora H. Does rapid microwave fixation improve immunohistochemistry? *Mod Pathol* 1990; 3:368–372.
12. Hopwood D, Coghill G, Ramsay J *et al.* Microwave fixation: its potential for routine techniques, histochemistry, immunocytochemistry and electron microscopy. *Histochem J* 1984; 16:1171–1191.
13. Login GR, Dvorak AM. Microwave fixation provides excellent preservation of tissue, cells and antigens for light and electron microscopy. *Histochem J* 1988; 20:373–387.
14. Morales AR, Nassiri M, Kanhoush R *et al.* Experience with an automated microwave-assisted rapid tissue processing method: validation of histologic quality and impact on the timeliness of diagnostic surgical pathology. *Am J Clin Pathol* 2004; 121:528–536.
15. Manne U, Myers RB, Srivastava S *et al.* Re: loss of tumor marker-immunostaining intensity on stored paraffin slides of breast cancer. *J Natl Cancer Inst* 1997; 89:585–586.
16. Shin HJ, Kalapurakal SK, Lee JJ *et al.* Comparison of p53 immunoreactivity in fresh-cut versus stored slides with and without microwave heating. *Mod Pathol* 1997; 10:224–230.
17. Cronin M, Pho M, Dutta D *et al.* Measurement of gene expression in archival paraffin-embedded tissues: development and performance of a 92-gene reverse transcriptase-polymerase chain reaction assay. *Am J Pathol* 2004; 164:35–42.
18. van den Broek LJ, van de Vijver MJ. Assessment of problems in diagnostic and research immunohistochemistry associated with epitope instability in stored paraffin sections. *Appl Immunohistochem Mol Morphol* 2000; 8:316–321.
19. Jacobs TW, Prioleau JE, Stillman IE *et al.* Loss of tumor marker-immunostaining intensity on stored paraffin slides of breast cancer. *J Natl Cancer Inst* 1996; 88:1054–1059.
20. Wester K, Wahlund E, Sundstrom C *et al.* Paraffin section storage and immunohistochemistry. Effects of time, temperature, fixation, and retrieval protocol with emphasis on p53 protein and MIB1 antigen. *Appl Immunohistochem Mol Morphol* 2000; 8:61–70.
21. DiVito KA, Charette LA, Rimm D *et al.* Long-term preservation of antigenicity on tissue microarrays. *Lab Invest* 2004; 84:1071–1078.
22. Shi SR, Shi Y, Taylor CR. Antigen retrieval immunohistochemistry: review and future prospects in research and diagnosis over two decades. *J Histochem Cytochem* 2011; 59:13–32.
23. Gown AM. Unmasking the mysteries of antigen or epitope retrieval and formalin fixation. *Am J Clin Pathol* 2004; 121:172–174.
24. Rakha EA, Reis-Filho JS, Baehner F *et al.* Breast cancer prognostic classification in the molecular era: the role of histological grade. *Breast Cancer Res* 2010; 12:207.
25. Burstein HJ, Winer EP. Refining therapy for human epidermal growth factor receptor 2-positive breast cancer: T stands for trastuzumab, tumor size, and treatment strategy. *J Clin Oncol* 2009; 27:5671–5673.
26. Paik S, Shak S, Tang G *et al.* A multigene assay to predict recurrence of tamoxifen-treated, node-negative breast cancer. *N Engl J Med* 2004; 351:2817–2826.
27. Paik S, Tang G, Shak S *et al.* Gene expression and benefit of chemotherapy in women with node-negative, estrogen receptor-positive breast cancer. *J Clin Oncol* 2006; 24:3726–3734.
28. Krag DN, Anderson SJ, Julian TB *et al.* Sentinel-lymph-node resection compared with conventional axillary-lymph-node dissection in clinically node-negative patients with breast cancer: overall survival findings from the NSABP B-32 randomised phase 3 trial. *Lancet Oncol* 2010; 11:927–933.
29. Giuliano AE, McCall L, Beitsch P *et al.* Locoregional recurrence after sentinel lymph node dissection with or without axillary dissection in patients with sentinel lymph node metastases: the American College of Surgeons Oncology Group Z0011 randomized trial. *Ann Surg* 2010; 252:426–432; discussion 432–423.

30. Edge SB, Compton CC. The American Joint Committee on Cancer: the 7th edition of the AJCC cancer staging manual and the future of TNM. *Ann Surg Oncol* 2010; 17:1471–1474.
31. Lee AH, Ellis IO. The Nottingham prognostic index for invasive carcinoma of the breast. *Pathol Oncol Res* 2008; 14:113–115.
32. Ravdin PM, Siminoff LA, Davis GJ *et al.* Computer program to assist in making decisions about adjuvant therapy for women with early breast cancer. *J Clin Oncol* 2001; 19:980–991.
33. Fisher ER, Wang J, Bryant J *et al.* Pathobiology of preoperative chemotherapy: findings from the National Surgical Adjuvant Breast and Bowel (NSABP) protocol B-18. *Cancer* 2002; 95:681–695.
34. Ogston KN, Miller ID, Payne S *et al.* A new histological grading system to assess response of breast cancers to primary chemotherapy: prognostic significance and survival. *Breast* 2003; 12:320–327.
35. Chevallier B, Roche H, Olivier JP *et al.* Inflammatory breast cancer. Pilot study of intensive induction chemotherapy (FEC-HD) results in a high histologic response rate. *Am J Clin Oncol* 1993; 16:223–228.
36. Sataloff DM, Mason BA, Prestipino AJ *et al.* Pathologic response to induction chemotherapy in locally advanced carcinoma of the breast: a determinant of outcome. *J Am Coll Surg* 1995; 180:297–306.
37. Symmans WF, Peintinger F, Hatzis C *et al.* Measurement of residual breast cancer burden to predict survival after neoadjuvant chemotherapy. *J Clin Oncol* 2007; 25:4414–4422.
38. Ellis MJ, Tao Y, Luo J *et al.* Outcome prediction for estrogen receptor-positive breast cancer based on postneoadjuvant endocrine therapy tumor characteristics. *J Natl Cancer Inst* 2008; 100:1380–1388.
39. Cheang MC, Treaba DO, Speers CH *et al.* Immunohistochemical detection using the new rabbit monoclonal antibody SP1 of estrogen receptor in breast cancer is superior to mouse monoclonal antibody 1D5 in predicting survival. *J Clin Oncol* 2006; 24:5637–5644.
40. Wolff AC, Hammond ME, Schwartz JN *et al.* American Society of Clinical Oncology/College of American Pathologists guideline recommendations for human epidermal growth factor receptor 2 testing in breast cancer. *J Clin Oncol* 2007; 25:118–145.
41. Perez EA, Dueck AC, McCullough AE *et al.* Predictability of adjuvant trastuzumab benefit in N9831 patients using the ASCO/CAP HER2-positivity criteria. *J Natl Cancer Inst* 2012; 104:159–162.
42. Paik S, Kim C, Wolmark N. HER2 status and benefit from adjuvant trastuzumab in breast cancer. *N Engl J Med* 2008; 358:1409–1411.
43. Dowsett M, Nielsen TO, A'Hern R *et al.* Assessment of Ki67 in breast cancer: recommendations from the International Ki67 in Breast Cancer working group. *J Natl Cancer Inst* 2011; 103:1656–1664.
44. Badve S, Dabbs DJ, Schnitt SJ *et al.* Basal-like and triple-negative breast cancers: a critical review with an emphasis on the implications for pathologists and oncologists. *Mod Pathol* 2011; 24:157–167.
45. Liedtke C, Broglio K, Moulder S *et al.* Prognostic impact of discordance between triple-receptor measurements in primary and recurrent breast cancer. *Ann Oncol* 2009; 20:1953–1958.
46. Gong Y, Han EY, Guo M *et al.* Stability of estrogen receptor status in breast carcinoma: a comparison between primary and metastatic tumors with regard to disease course and intervening systemic therapy. *Cancer* 2011; 117:705–713.
47. Perou CM, Sorlie T, Eisen MB *et al.* Molecular portraits of human breast tumours. *Nature* 2000; 406:747–752.
48. Sorlie T, Tibshirani R, Parker J *et al.* Repeated observation of breast tumor subtypes in independent gene expression data sets. *Proc Natl Acad Sci USA* 2003; 100:8418–8423.
49. Weigelt B, Mackay A, A'Hern R *et al.* Breast cancer molecular profiling with single sample predictors: a retrospective analysis. *Lancet Oncol* 2010; 11:339–349.
50. Parker JS, Mullins M, Cheang MC *et al.* Supervised risk predictor of breast cancer based on intrinsic subtypes. *J Clin Oncol* 2009; 27:1160–1167.
51 Dowsett M, Lopez-Knowles E, Sidhu K *et al.* Comparison of PAM50 risk of recurrence (ROR) score with Onco*type* DX and IHC4 for predicting residual risk of RFS and distant-(D)RFS after endocrine therapy: a TransATAC study. *Cancer Research* 2012; 71:S4–5.
52. van de Vijver MJ, He YD, van't Veer LJ *et al.* A gene-expression signature as a predictor of survival in breast cancer. *N Engl J Med* 2002; 347:1999–2009.
53. van't Veer LJ, Dai H, van de Vijver MJ *et al.* Gene expression profiling predicts clinical outcome of breast cancer. *Nature* 2002; 415:530–536.
54. Cardoso F, Piccart-Gebhart M, Van't Veer L *et al.* The MINDACT trial: the first prospective clinical validation of a genomic tool. *Mol Oncol* 2007; 1:246–251.
55. Sparano JA. TAILORx: trial assigning individualized options for treatment (Rx). *Clin Breast Cancer* 2006; 7:347–350.

56. Zujewski JA, Kamin L. Trial assessing individualized options for treatment for breast cancer: the TAILORx trial. *Future Oncol* 2008; 4:603–610.
57. Shah SP, Roth A, Goya R *et al.* The clonal and mutational evolution spectrum of primary triple-negative breast cancers. *Nature* 2012; 486:395–399.
58. Stephens PJ, Tarpey PS, Davies H *et al.* The landscape of cancer genes and mutational processes in breast cancer. *Nature* 2012; 486:400–404.
59. Ellis MJ, Ding L, Shen D *et al.* Whole-genome analysis informs breast cancer response to aromatase inhibition. *Nature* 2012; 486:353–360.
60. Banerji S, Cibulskis K, Rangel-Escareno C *et al.* Sequence analysis of mutations and translocations across breast cancer subtypes. *Nature* 2012; 486:405–409.
61. Curtis C, Shah SP, Chin SF *et al.* The genomic and transcriptomic architecture of 2,000 breast tumours reveals novel subgroups. *Nature* 2012; 486:346–352.
62. Lehmann BD, Bauer JA, Chen X *et al.* Identification of human triple-negative breast cancer subtypes and preclinical models for selection of targeted therapies. *J Clin Invest* 2011; 121:2750–2767.
63. Weigelt B, Warne PH, Downward J. PIK3CA mutation, but not PTEN loss of function, determines the sensitivity of breast cancer cells to mTOR inhibitory drugs. *Oncogene* 2011; 30:3222–3233.
64. Heiser LM, Wang NJ, Talcott CL *et al.* Integrated analysis of breast cancer cell lines reveals unique signaling pathways. *Genome Biol* 2009; 10:R31.
65. Janku F, Wheler JJ, Westin SN *et al.* PI3K/AKT/mTOR inhibitors in patients with breast and gynecologic malignancies harboring PIK3CA mutations. *J Clin Oncol* 2012; 30:777–782.
66. Brough R, Frankum JR, Sims D *et al.* Functional viability profiles of breast cancer. *Cancer Discov* 2011; 1:260–273.
67. Robertson FM (ed.) Gene amplification of anaplastic lymphoma kinase in inflammatory breast cancer. *Molecular Targets and Cancer Therapeutics*; 2011; San Francisco: Proceedings of the AACR-NCI-EORTC International Conference.
68. Tang G, Cuzick J, Costantino JP *et al.* Risk of recurrence and chemotherapy benefit for patients with node-negative, estrogen receptor-positive breast cancer: recurrence score alone and integrated with pathologic and clinical factors. *J Clin Oncol* 2011; 29:4365–4372.

3

Chemoprevention of breast cancer

D. L. Wickerham

INTRODUCTION

The American Cancer Society estimated that there were 226 870 new cases of invasive breast cancer diagnosed in the United States in 2012 and more than 1 million new cases worldwide [1]. Despite newer treatments and improvements in screening, more than 39 000 will die from this disease each year in the United States. Breast cancer remains a major health issue for all women, and, therefore, the concept of prevention is an attractive addition to screening and treatment.

Although some factors that appear to contribute to breast cancer risk, such as postmenopausal obesity, dietary fat intake, and alcohol consumption, may be modifiable, the factors that put a woman at greatest risk – gender, age, and family history [2] – are not amenable to lifestyle modifications. Prophylactic mastectomy is an effective strategy for some women at high risk for the disease, but it is a drastic and irreversible choice [3].

This chapter will focus on the chemoprevention of breast cancer using targeted agents. Hong and Sporn [4] have defined chemoprevention as: '*the use of pharmacologic or natural agents that inhibit the development of invasive cancer either by blocking the DNA damage that initiates carcinogenesis or by arresting or reversing the progression of premalignant cells in which such damage has already occurred*' (Box 3.1).

Breast cancer chemoprevention has already demonstrated substantial clinical success [5–8]. Hormones appear to play a significant role in the development of this disease, and current chemoprevention strategies have targeted hormonally responsive breast cancers.

THERAPIES IN CURRENT USE IN BREAST CANCER PREVENTION

The targeted chemoprevention agent with the greatest clinical use to date is the selective estrogen receptor modulator (SERM) tamoxifen. This drug is a well-established treatment for receptor-positive breast cancer and is among the most commonly prescribed breast cancer drugs in the world. It has a demonstrated effectiveness in reducing the risk of recurrence and reducing the risk of death from breast cancer [9]. Tamoxifen also has a well-defined safety profile and the added benefits that it helps maintain bone density in postmenopausal women and has a positive impact on lipid profiles. In the trials that demonstrated tamoxifen to be an effective treatment for breast cancer, there was also a substantial reduction in new primary cancers of the opposite breast that persisted for up to 15 years [10–13].

D. Lawrence Wickerham, MD, National Surgical Adjuvant Breast and Bowel Project, Pittsburgh, Pennsylvania, USA.

Box 3.1 Definition of chemoprevention

"Chemoprevention is the use of pharmacologic or natural agents that inhibit the development of invasive cancer either by blocking the DNA damage that initiates carcinogenesis or by arresting or reversing the progression of premalignant cells in which such damage has already occurred."

From: Hong WK, Sporn MB [4]

THE NSABP BREAST CANCER PREVENTION TRIAL

The treatment trial findings and extensive laboratory data demonstrating tamoxifen's chemopreventative properties led to the initial randomized breast cancer prevention trials [14–20] (Figure 3.1). The largest of these was the NSABP Breast Cancer Prevention Trial, P-1, which randomly assigned more than 13 000 women in a double-blind fashion to receive 20 mg of tamoxifen daily or placebo for a 5-year period.

Eligible participants in this study were women at increased risk of developing breast cancer, risk being defined as:

1. Being at least 60 years of age; or
2. Having a history of lobular carcinoma *in situ* (LCIS); or
3. Having a 5-year projected breast cancer risk of at least 1.66% as determined by the modified Gail Model [5].

Participants were ineligible if they had a history of deep vein thrombosis (DVT) or pulmonary emboli or if they were taking hormone replacement therapy, oral contraceptives, or androgens for at least 3 months before random assignment. The trial participants were also required not to use these hormones during the course of the study. The primary endpoint of the trial was the incidence of invasive breast cancer, but secondary endpoints included all invasive cancers, non-invasive breast and endometrial cancers, cardiac events, fractures of the hip, spine, or Colles' fractures of the wrist, and death from any cause. There was also a formal quality-of-life (QOL) evaluation at entry, at 3 months, at 6 months, and at each 6-month period thereafter.

With an average follow-up of approximately 4 years, there was a statistically significant 49% reduction in invasive breast cancers in favor of the tamoxifen-treated women [5]. The relative risk (RR) comparing tamoxifen to placebo was 0.51, with a 95% confidence interval (CI) of 0.39–0.66. The rate of non-invasive breast cancers (LCIS and ductal carcinoma *in situ* [DCIS] combined) was reduced by a similar magnitude. The reduction of invasive breast cancer appeared to be only in estrogen-receptor-positive disease, with a 69% reduction of the incidence in these patients; there was no difference between the treatment groups in terms of incidence of estrogen-receptor-negative disease.

As noted above, there were three sites included in the P-1 trial as endpoints for markers of osteoporotic fractures: fractures of the hip, spine, and Colles' fractures of the wrist. There was a 45% reduction in the number of these fractures with tamoxifen, 79 in the placebo group and 49 in the tamoxifen group.

Since tamoxifen treatment was known to reduce blood lipids, specific cardiovascular endpoints were included in the P-1 trial to evaluate whether or not tamoxifen could reduce the risk of myocardial infarction and severe angina or acute ischemic syndrome. No significant reduction was evident: there were 28 cases of myocardial infarction in the placebo-treated group and 31 in the tamoxifen-treated group (RR 1.11; 95% CI 0.65–1.92). There also were no statistically significant differences in the other two cardiac disease endpoints.

Studies evaluating the use of tamoxifen in the treatment of invasive breast cancer have shown an association between therapy and an increase in the risk of endometrial cancer and

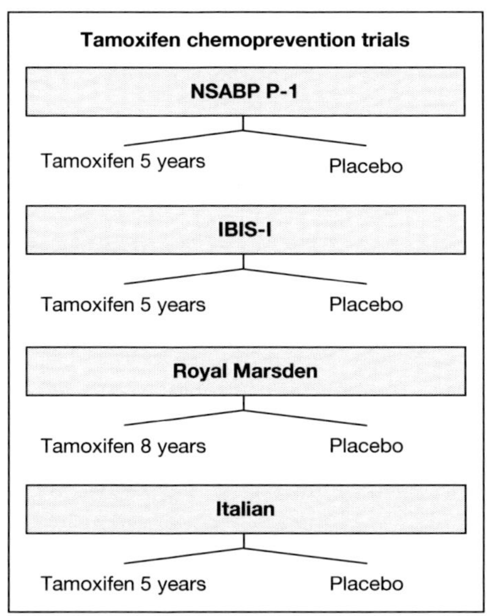

Figure 3.1 Large randomized breast cancer prevention trials.

thromboembolic events. We saw these elevated risks in the P-1 trial as well: the RR for endometrial adenocarcinoma was 2.53 (95% CI 1.35–4.97), with 15 cases occurring in the placebo group compared to 36 in the tamoxifen group. This increased risk occurred predominantly among those 50 years of age or older at the time of random assignment. The endometrial cancers that developed in women who received tamoxifen did not appear to be different in terms of pathology or pathogenicity from those that occurred in the placebo-treated women. Although rare, the risk of uterine sarcoma also appeared to be elevated among those who received tamoxifen [21]. The most recent follow-up data from the P-1 trial indicate there were four cases of uterine sarcoma reported among the women who received tamoxifen and one in the placebo group (RR 3.98; 95% CI 0.39–195.94). With regard to thromboembolic events associated with tamoxifen use, the risk for these appears to be similar in magnitude to that of postmenopausal women who take estrogen replacement therapy. In the P-1 trial there was a 60% increase in the risk of DVT (RR 1.60; 95% CI 0.91–2.86), with 22 cases occurring in the placebo group and 35 in the tamoxifen group. The risk of pulmonary embolism was also increased threefold (RR 3.01; 95% CI 1.15–9.27), with 6 and 18 cases occurring in the placebo and tamoxifen groups, respectively. Although not statistically significant, there also appeared to be an increased risk of stroke of about 59% (RR 1.59; 95% CI 0.93–2.77). There were 24 strokes among women in the placebo group and 38 in the tamoxifen group. As with endometrial cancer, the increased risk of thromboembolic events occurred predominantly in women 50 years of age or older at the time of random assignment. One theory regarding the association of tamoxifen and thromboembolic risk is that tamoxifen causes blood clotting in those with gene mutations associated with serum factors that increase the likelihood of clotting disorders such as Factor V Leiden or prothrombin 20210A [22]. However, an interaction of tamoxifen with these types of mutations is not evident. Although the risk of thromboembolic events does appear to be elevated in women who have these mutations, in the P-1 trial there was no difference in the magnitude of such risk between the placebo and tamoxifen groups [22].

The P-1 trial also analyzed the effects of tamoxifen on several QOL endpoints [23]. There were no differences between the tamoxifen and the placebo groups in terms of scoring on the Center for Epidemiologic Studies-Depression Scale (CES-D), in the Medical Outcomes Study (MOS) SF-36 summary physical and mental scores, or on numerous subscales that included measurements of physical functioning, bodily pain, vitality, mental health, general health perception, social functioning, role-physical or role-emotional. Despite several reports in the literature of a possible relationship between tamoxifen use and depression [24], data from the P-1 trial did not support this finding: when stratified by depression risk (based on conditions reported at baseline) and the duration of follow-up, there was no evidence to suggest that tamoxifen increased the rate of depression.

Weight gain is another effect that has been anecdotally associated with tamoxifen, but evidence from the P-1 trial did not statistically support such an association, and we found that the proportion of women who reported weight *loss* during the first 3 years of treatment was slightly higher in the tamoxifen group (44.9%) than in the placebo group (42.2%). Several symptoms were associated with tamoxifen use, including vasomotor effects (hot flashes, night sweats, cold sweats) and gynecological symptoms (vaginal dryness, vaginal discharge, and vaginal itching).

Data about the use of tamoxifen in women with *BRCA1* or *BRCA2* inherited mutations are very limited, and definitive statements about the effectiveness of tamoxifen in such patients is not currently available. King and colleagues [25] evaluated 288 breast cancer patients in the P-1 trial and identified only 19 women with inherited *BRCA1* or *BRCA2* mutations. Tamoxifen reduced the breast cancer incidence among the *BRCA2* carriers by 62% (RR 0.38; 95% CI 0.06–1.56), but a reduction was not noted in women with *BRCA1* mutations (RR 1.67; 95% CI 0.32–10.70). Narod and colleagues [26] published a matched-case controlled study that demonstrated significant protection against contralateral breast cancer in women with known *BRCA1* mutations who developed invasive breast cancer and were treated with tamoxifen (odds ratio [OR] 0.38; 95% CI 0.19–0.74). A lesser effect was seen in women with *BRCA2* mutations (OR 0.62; 95% CI 0.20–1.50). The papers together suggest women with *BRCA1* or *BRCA2* mutations who have or will develop ER-positive breast cancer are potential candidates for tamoxifen therapy, but at the present time it is not possible to determine which women with *BRCA1* or *BRCA2* mutations will develop ER-positive disease.

Women with a biopsy-proven history of LCIS or atypical hyperplasia of the breast have a substantially increased 5-year risk of developing breast cancer, and this is reflected in their Gail scores. In the P-1 trial, the annual breast cancer rate per 1000 women in the placebo arm for those with a history of LCIS at the time of entry was 12.99 and for those with a prior history of atypical hyperplasia it was 10.11. Both groups showed a substantial benefit from tamoxifen, with a 56% reduction of invasive breast cancer in the women with LCIS and an 86% reduction in those with atypical hyperplasia.

ADDITIONAL TAMOXIFEN PREVENTION TRIALS

Several additional tamoxifen prevention trials have been carried out. These were of different sizes, had slightly different designs, and produced variable results. The International Breast Cancer Intervention Study (IBIS-I) studied 7145 women aged 35–70 years who were at increased risk for breast cancer and randomly assigned them to receive tamoxifen 20 mg/day or placebo for 5 years [6]. The initial results, published in 2002 with 49 months of median follow-up, demonstrated that tamoxifen reduced the risk of ER-positive breast cancer by 31%. Updated results demonstrate that these benefits persist for at least 10 years [27].

The Royal Marsden Trial [28] began in 1986 as a pilot trial to evaluate the feasibility of a tamoxifen prevention trial. Between 1986 and 1996, 2471 eligible participants entered the study and were assigned to receive either tamoxifen 20 mg/day or placebo for an 8-year period. The first analysis reported in 1998 found no reduction in breast cancer incidence, but a more recent paper [29] with a median of 13 years of follow-up shows a statistically significant reduction in ER-positive breast cancer.

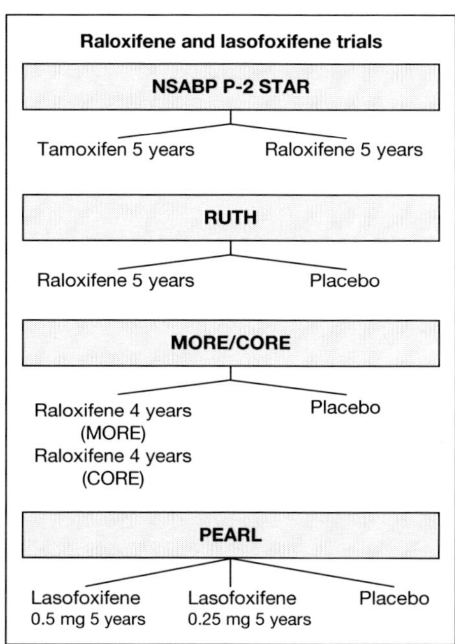

Figure 3.2 Raloxifene and lasofoxifene trials in breast cancer prevention and osteoporotic fracture.

The Italian Tamoxifen Prevention Study [30] randomly assigned 5408 women aged 35–70 years to receive tamoxifen or placebo, but this study was not restricted to women at increased risk of breast cancer. The original sample size was substantially larger, but accrual was halted by the data and safety monitoring committee overseeing the study, due in part to poor adherence; 26% of the women discontinued treatment within the first year. The initial published results failed to demonstrate an overall benefit for tamoxifen, but in the subset of 1580 women who used estrogen replacement therapy at some point during the study, there were 23 breast cancers, 17 in the placebo group and six in the tamoxifen group (hazard ratio [HR] 0.35; 95% CI 0.14–0.89) [31]. This finding led to the HRT Opposed to low-dose Tamoxifen (HOT Study) [32] to evaluate tamoxifen 5 mg/day in women taking hormone replacement therapy.

An overview of the tamoxifen prevention trials was published in 2003 and reported a 37% decrease in invasive breast cancer in the combined tamoxifen treatment groups [7]. Data are currently being analyzed for an update of the overview.

RALOXIFENE STUDIES IN BREAST CANCER REDUCTION AND OSTEOPOROTIC FRACTURE (FIGURE 3.2)

Raloxifene is a second-generation benzothiophene SERM that has been available for more than a decade for the treatment and prevention of osteoporosis in postmenopausal women. The drug competes with estrogen at the estrogen-receptor and binds to both ER Alpha and ER Beta [33–35]. It is an estrogen agonist in bone and an estrogen antagonist in the uterus and breast. The estrogen agonist effects on breast tissue are thought to be the result of blocking coactivator binding to the activating function-2 domain of the estrogen-receptor, which in turn blocks transcription of ER-regulated genes. Raloxifene may have additional effects on breast tissue other than its direct effects at the estrogen-receptor, including effects on estrogen bioavailability, effects on insulin-like growth factors, and a role in estrogen-induced biosynthesis [36]. Preclinical models show that raloxifene has prevented or inhibited the growth of breast cancer cells *in vitro* and tumors [37–41] in animal models.

Therapeutic clinical efficacy

Raloxifene was initially evaluated as a possible treatment for breast cancer. The results showed limited effectiveness, and further examination of its use in breast cancer treatment was discontinued.

Raloxifene has well-established favorable effects on bone metabolism in postmenopausal women [42, 43]. At 60 mg/day, this drug has been shown to preserve or increase bone mineral density (BMD) [44], to decrease markers of bone turnover [45], and to be associated with a positive shift in calcium balance [46].

The Multiple Outcomes of Raloxifene Evaluation (MORE) Study

The pivotal raloxifene study that led to its approval by the US Food and Drug Administration (FDA) was the MORE Study. The MORE trial randomly assigned 7705 postmenopausal women with osteoporosis to receive oral raloxifene, 60 mg/day ($n = 2557$), raloxifene 120 mg/day ($n = 2572$), or placebo ($n = 2576$) [47]. The participants also received daily supplements of calcium 500 mg/day and Vitamin D 400–600 I.U. The study was designed for 3 years, but was later extended to 4 years [48, 49]. The primary objective of this double-blind international trial was to evaluate the effects of raloxifene compared to placebo on the incidence of vertebral fractures and BMD in this population of women. Secondary endpoints included the effect of raloxifene on breast cancer incidence. Participants in MORE were not selected or prospectively evaluated for their breast cancer risk. Women with osteoporosis generally have a lower risk of breast cancer that corresponds to their lower levels of estradiol [50, 51].

The MORE results demonstrated a significant reduction in vertebral fractures in the raloxifene-treated women compared to those in the placebo group, but the incidence of non-vertebral fractures was not significantly different [47]. The risk of invasive breast cancer was reduced in the raloxifene groups by 76% after 3 years (RR 0.24; 95% CI 0.13–0.44) and by 72% after 4 years (RR 0.28; 95% CI 0.17–0.46). As with tamoxifen, this benefit was specific to receptor-positive (ER+) invasive breast cancers, which were reduced by 84%, and there was a non-significant change in estrogen-receptor-negative (ER–) disease. In addition, no significant differences were noted between the two raloxifene groups for either fracture or breast cancer prevention. An increased risk of venous thromboembolic events, including DVT and pulmonary embolism (PE), was identified (RR 3.1; 95% CI 1.5–6.2), but, unlike tamoxifen, with raloxifene there was no difference in the incidence of endometrial cancer.

The Continuing Outcomes Relevant to Evista (CORE) Trial

The CORE trial [52] was a double-blinded, placebo-controlled study that evaluated the efficacy of an additional 4 years of raloxifene compared to placebo in reducing the risk of invasive breast cancer in women who had participated in the MORE trial. Women entering CORE who received raloxifene in MORE (either 60 mg/day or 120 mg/day) were given raloxifene 60 mg/day, and the MORE placebo-treated women continued to receive placebo in CORE. The primary breast cancer analysis included 3996 patients who had completed MORE and agreed to enter CORE, plus 1217 patients who were still participating in MORE when CORE began and contributed data. Secondary endpoints in the CORE study included the incidence of ER+ breast cancer and the incidence of invasive breast cancer from the start of the MORE trial to the end of the CORE trial. The incidence of invasive breast cancer was reduced by 59% (HR 0.41; 95% CI 0.24–0.71) in women in the raloxifene-treated group compared to those in the placebo group, and there was a 66% reduction in ER-positive invasive breast cancer (HR 0.24; 95% CI 0.18–0.66). Over the 8 years of both trials, the incidence of invasive breast cancer was reduced by 66% (HR 0.34; 95% CI 0.22–0.50), and no new safety concerns related to raloxifene therapy were identified.

The Raloxifene Use for the Heart (RUTH) Trial

Raloxifene has been shown to have favorable effects on serum lipid levels [45] in postmenopausal women, with statistically significant reductions in total cholesterol and low-density lipoprotein (LDL) cholesterol levels [53], but it does not appear to significantly alter high-density lipoprotein cholesterol or triglyceride levels [54, 55]. The Raloxifene Use for the Heart (RUTH) trial was designed to follow-up on these favorable effects on markers of cardiovascular risk. The study compared the effects of raloxifene (60 mg/day) to placebo on the incidence of coronary events and invasive breast cancer in 10 101 postmenopausal women at increased risk for major coronary events [56]. The mean age of the women in this trial was 67.5 years; 84% were white and 41% had a modified 5-year Gail score of 1.67% or greater. At a median follow-up of 5.6 years, there was no significant difference between the raloxifene and placebo groups for coronary events in the RUTH trial. The rate of invasive breast cancer was reduced by 44% in the raloxifene group (1.5/1000 women years in the raloxifene group, compared to 2.7/1000 women years in the placebo group). As in the MORE and CORE studies, the benefit was seen in ER-positive cancer (0.9 vs. 2.1/1000 women years) but not in ER-negative cancers (0.5 vs. 0.3/1000 women years). The rate of non-invasive breast cancer (0.4 vs. 0.2/1000 women years) was not significantly different between the raloxifene and placebo groups (HR 2.17; 95% CI 0.75–6.24). Mortality rates overall did not differ between the raloxifene and placebo recipients (20.7 vs. 22.5 deaths/1000 women years). The rate of stroke was not different between the groups (9.5 raloxifene vs. 8.6 placebo cases/1000 women years), but the rate of death from stroke was higher in the raloxifene group (2.2 vs. 1.5 deaths/1000 women years). Increases in stroke or fatal strokes were not seen in MORE nor in a post hoc subgroup analysis of MORE women with increased cardiovascular risk at baseline ($n = 1035$). However, the US prescribing information does contain a black box to consider the risk/benefit for raloxifene in women at increased risk for stroke.

The NSABP Study of Tamoxifen and Raloxifene (STAR) (P-2)

The results of NSABP's P-1 trial were initially published in 1998 and demonstrated that tamoxifen could reduce the incidence of breast cancer by up to 50% in a population of otherwise healthy women at increased risk for the future development of the disease [5]. With the results of the various raloxifene studies demonstrating that in a population of women not selected for their breast cancer risk there was an impressive reduction in the relative risk of breast cancer, the Study of Tamoxifen and Raloxifene (STAR) trial was the next logical step.

This study was a double-blinded, randomized clinical trial that entered 19 747 postmenopausal women who were at least 35 years of age and had a history of LCIS treated by local excision alone or a modified Gail score demonstrating a 5-year risk for invasive breast cancer of at least 1.66% [8]. Women were assigned to take either tamoxifen 20 mg/day plus a placebo, or raloxifene 60 mg/day plus a placebo, for a 5-year period. The primary endpoint of the trial was the development of invasive breast cancer. Secondary endpoints included non-invasive breast cancer, uterine malignancy, thromboembolic events, fractures, cataracts, QOL, and death. To minimize the risk of stroke or thromboembolic events, eligible participants could not have a history of stroke, transient ischemic attack (TIA), PE, DVT, uncontrolled diabetes, uncontrolled hypertension, or uncontrolled atrial fibrillation.

The mean age of the participants, all of whom were postmenopausal, was 58.5 years, and the mean 5-year risk of developing invasive breast cancer based on the modified Gail score was 4.03%. The projected lifetime risk to these women to 80 years of age was 16%. Over 70% of the women entering the trial had one or more first-degree female relative with breast cancer, and more than 9% reported a personal history of LCIS. In addition, over 22% had had a breast biopsy prior to enrolment that demonstrated either atypical ductal (ADH) or atypical lobular hyperplasia (ALH). Just over 50% of the participants reported having undergone a hysterectomy, with or without oopherectomy, before random assignment.

The initial published results of the STAR trial showed that 163 of the women assigned to tamoxifen and 168 of those assigned to raloxifene had developed an invasive breast cancer, demonstrating that there was no difference in the effects of tamoxifen and raloxifene on the incidence of invasive breast cancer. The rate per 1000 women years was 4.3 in the tamoxifen group and 4.4 in the raloxifene group (RR 1.02; 95% CI 0.82–1.28). Although there was no placebo-alone group in this trial, the Gail model scores of the women who entered the trial allow us to estimate the number of invasive breast cancers that would have occurred in an untreated group and demonstrate that there was about a 47% reduction in incidence of invasive breast cancer. The cumulative incidence of invasive breast cancer at 72 months for the two treatment groups was 25.1 for the tamoxifen group and 24.8 for the raloxifene group ($P=0.83$). When the treatment groups were compared by baseline characteristics of age, history of LCIS or atypical hyperplasia, Gail score, and number of first-degree relatives with breast cancer, the pattern of no differential effect by treatment group remained consistent, and none of the relative risks in the subsets were statistically significant. The characteristics of the invasive breast cancers showed no differences between the treatment groups with regard to distribution by tumor size, nodal status, or estrogen-receptor level.

Raloxifene did not appear to be as effective as tamoxifen in reducing the incidence of non-invasive breast cancers (LCIS or DCIS), although the difference did not reach statistical significance. There were 57 cases of non-invasive breast cancer among the women assigned to tamoxifen and 80 among women who took raloxifene (1.51/1000 women assigned to tamoxifen and 2.1/1000 women assigned to raloxifene [RR 1.40; 95% CI 0.98–2.00]). The cumulative incidence through 6 years was 8.1/1000 in the tamoxifen group and 11.6/1000 in the raloxifene group ($P=0.052$). Recall that the previous P-1 tamoxifen/placebo trial had demonstrated a nearly 50% reduction in non-invasive breast cancers in favor of the tamoxifen-treated women [5].

More uterine malignancies occurred in the tamoxifen-treated women than in those treated with raloxifene, but the difference was not statistically significant at the time of the original analysis. There were 36 cases in the tamoxifen group and 23 cases in the raloxifene group, with an annual incidence rate of 1.99/1000 and 1.25/1000, respectively (RR 0.63; 95% CI 0.35–1.08). Uterine hyperplasia with and without atypia was significantly less common in the raloxifene-treated group. There were also significantly fewer hysterectomies performed for non-malignant indications in the raloxifene group (244 tamoxifen; 111 raloxifene [RR 0.39; 95% CI 0.30–0.50]). There were no statistically significant differences between the treatment groups in regard to other malignancies.

No statistically significant differences were noted between the two groups relative to the incidence of ischemic heart disease, TIA, stroke, or fractures. Significantly fewer thromboembolic events (DVT or PE) occurred in the raloxifene-treated group. Fewer women on raloxifene developed cataracts during treatment, and fewer underwent surgical removal of those cataracts.

Mortality in the two groups was similar, with 101 deaths in those assigned to tamoxifen and 96 deaths in those assigned to raloxifene, resulting in a rate of 2.64/1000 and 2.49/1000 respectively (RR 0.94; 95% CI 0.71–1.26). The distribution by cause of death did not differ by treatment.

The STAR results were updated with a median of 81 months of follow-up, which represents 5 years of SERM treatment and approximately an additional 2 years of follow-up [57]. Raloxifene retained 76% of the effectiveness of tamoxifen in preventing invasive disease, but with the additional data tamoxifen was shown to be superior statistically (RR 1.24; 95% CI 1.05–1.47). Compared with the initial results, the RR for non-invasive cancer narrowed (RR 1.22; 95% CI 0.95–1.59). There continued to be no significant mortality differences, and raloxifene continued to be less toxic. The incidence of invasive uterine cancer was significantly lower in the raloxifene group ($P = 0.003$). The average annual incidence rate of uterine hyperplasia was five times higher in the tamoxifen group, and the number of hysterectomies performed for benign disease was more than double that performed in the raloxifene group. Neither tamoxifen nor raloxifene conferred a higher relative risk for ischemic heart disease or stroke, irrespective of coronary heart disease (CHD). Tamoxifen was associated with a significantly higher RR of thromboembolic events, particularly in women with pre-existing CHD.[1]

Why do we see an apparent diminution in raloxifene's benefits with the prolonged follow-up? When the STAR results were first published, participants were notified of their treatment assignment, and those women who had not yet completed 5 years of tamoxifen were offered the opportunity to cross over to raloxifene for the remainder of the 5 years. Relatively few patients selected this option, and crossover is unlikely to fully explain the updated results. Adherence to protocol medication or drop-offs are also unlikely to explain the findings. Adherence, as measured by pill counts, was similar in the two groups, and protocol medication drop-off rates were higher in the tamoxifen group (38% vs. 27.4%).

The rate-limiting step of tamoxifen metabolism to its active metabolite is the CYP2D6-medicated oxidation of N-desmethyl tamoxifen [58–59], and common genetic variations in CYP2D6 as well as drug-induced inhibition of CYP2D6 activity reduce endoxifen concentrations [60]. Raloxifene is not metabolized in this manner and is not known to be impacted by the CYP2D6 genotype. A nested case-control study of postmenopausal women in STAR and P-1 who developed breast cancer while on either tamoxifen or raloxifene demonstrated that alterations in CYP2D6 metabolism are not associated with either tamoxifen or raloxifene efficacy [61]. Raloxifene may simply be less potent than tamoxifen. Raloxifene was originally developed as a drug to treat breast cancer, and it was less effective than tamoxifen in that setting as well [62]. However, laboratory studies demonstrate that the antitumor actions of raloxifene and other hydroxylated SERMs depend on the duration of therapy. The 5-year duration of therapy in STAR was a carry-over from the P-1 study of tamoxifen versus placebo. Raloxifene in the treatment or prevention of osteoporosis can be given for an indefinite period. In the combined MORE and CORE trials, which involved as much as 8 years of raloxifene therapy, a 66% reduction in the incidence of breast cancer was seen in the raloxifene-treated group compared to placebo (HR 0.34; 95% CI 0.22–0.50). Continuing raloxifene therapy beyond 5 years might be an approach to maintain its full chemopreventive activity. The superiority of 5 years of tamoxifen over raloxifene in reducing breast cancer risk comes with a cost: more endometrial cancers, hysterectomies for benign disease, thromboembolic events, and cataracts. Both drugs remain acceptable options for postmenopausal women wishing to reduce their risk of breast cancer. Risk/benefit assessment may impact the drug choice for individual patients, addressed in an article by Friedman and colleagues [63].

The STAR trial included a formal QOL assessment in a subset of 1983 participants who submitted a 36-item symptom checklist, a MOS short form health survey (SF-36), the CES-D, and the MOS sexual activity questionnaire [64]. These questionnaires were administered before treatment, every 6 months for 60 months, and at 72 months. No significant differences existed between the tamoxifen and raloxifene groups in patient-reported outcomes for over-

[1] Reis S *et al. Cardiovascular effects of tamoxifen in women with and without heart disease: The National Surgical Adjuvant Breast and Bowel Project Study of Tamoxifen and Raloxifene (STAR) P-2 Trial*. Manuscript in progress.

all physical health, mental health, and depression, although the tamoxifen group reported better sexual function. Of the women in the symptom assessment analyses, the 9769 in the raloxifene group reported greater mean symptom severity over 60 months of assessments than did the 9743 in the tamoxifen group for musculoskeletal problems, dyspareunia, and weight gain. The women in the tamoxifen group reported greater mean symptom severity for gynecologic problems, vasomotor symptoms, leg cramps, and bladder control symptoms. It is important to point out that the mean symptom severity was low among these postmenopausal women, and the significant differences were small relative to established standards for minimal clinically important differences in these various scales.

The data from the MORE, CORE, RUTH, and STAR trials resulted in approval of raloxifene by the US FDA for the reduction in risk of invasive breast cancer in postmenopausal women with osteoporosis and reduction in risk of invasive breast cancer in postmenopausal women at high risk of invasive breast cancer. No data are currently available on the use of raloxifene in patients with the inherited mutations such as BRCA1 and 2 abnormalities, nor was raloxifene approved for women with a previous invasive breast cancer or for the treatment of invasive breast cancer. However, raloxifene's approval does give an important new option to postmenopausal women beyond that of tamoxifen, one that avoids an excess of endometrial cancers and reduces the risk of thromboembolic events. Unlike tamoxifen, raloxifene is already used widely by primary care physicians for the treatment and prevention of osteoporosis. Although the risk reduction is restricted to ER-positive breast cancers, these are the majority of breast cancers that occur, and this represents an important step in breast cancer chemoprevention. Raloxifene use is restricted to postmenopausal women because there are few data on its safety or efficacy in premenopausal women.

ADDITIONAL SERMS

There are at least two additional SERMs in development that may prove to be of value in breast cancer chemoprevention. The first is lasofoxifene. The results of the Postmenopausal Evaluation and Risk-Reduction with Lasofoxifene (PEARL) Study were presented at the 2008 San Antonio Breast Cancer Symposium [65]. This study evaluated 8556 postmenopausal women with osteoporosis and assigned them to receive either placebo or lasofoxifene at 0.25 mg/day or 0.5 mg/day. For all invasive breast cancers, there were 20 cases in the placebo group, 16 in the 0.25 mg/day lasofoxifene group (HR 0.79; 95% CI 0.41–1.52), and three in the 0.5 mg/day group (HR 0.15; 95% CI 0.04–0.50). Lasofoxifene also reduced the incidence of vertebral and non-vertebral fractures but increased the risk of venus thromboembolic events, although not stroke, endometrial cancer, or endometrial hyperplasia. Endometrial hypertrophy, uterine polyps, and fibroids were more common in the lasofoxifene-treated women.

The other SERM being developed was arzoxifene. The Generations trial is a multi-center placebo-controlled, double-blind trial that compared arzoxifene 20 mg/day and placebo in 9354 postmenopausal women with osteoporosis or low bone mass.[2] After 48 months of follow-up, 53 breast cancers had occurred in the placebo group and 22 in the arzoxifene group (HR 0.41; 95% CI 0.25–0.68; $P=0.001$). As with other SERMs, the benefit in breast cancer risk reduction was limited to ER-positive disease, with 30 invasive ER-positive cases in the placebo group and 9 in the arzoxifene group (HR 0.30; 95% CI 0.14–0.63; $P=0.001$). Although the results demonstrate that arzoxifene is effective in reducing breast cancer risk, its antifracture efficacy compared to other osteoporosis treatments was not sufficient to justify further clinical development of the drug.

[2] Powles TJ, Diem SJ, Fabian CJ *et al. Breast cancer incidence in postmenopausal women with osteoporosis or low bone mass using arzoxifene*. Manuscript in progress.

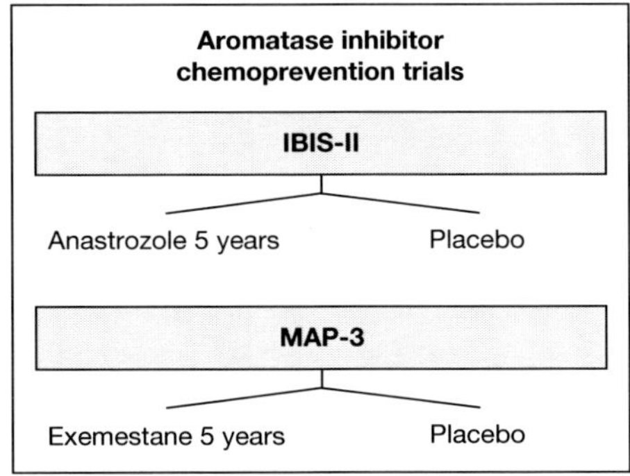

Figure 3.3 Trials of aromatase inhibitors in breast cancer prevention.

AROMATASE INHIBITORS

In postmenopausal women, aromatase inhibitors (AIs) block the production of estrogens in extra-gonadal peripheral tissues. Circulatory estrogen levels are dramatically reduced, and aromatase activity in the breast may also be affected. High circulatory estrogen levels as well as high aromatase levels in breast tissue have been linked to an increased breast cancer risk [66].

The development of so-called third-generation selective AIs has already had a profound impact on the adjuvant treatment of postmenopausal women with receptor-positive breast cancer. Studies in advanced disease have shown that these newer AIs are as good as, or better than, the standard hormonal therapies [67–71]. In adjuvant trials of various design, these AIs result in improved disease-free survival (DFS) and are associated with fewer life-threatening side-effects than is tamoxifen [72–76]. However, the use of AIs does frequently result in arthralgias/myalgias and bone loss, which may prove to be a barrier to their use for prevention. Relative to breast cancer prevention, the women in these adjuvant trials who received AIs had a decrease in new primary breast cancers of the opposite breast compared to tamoxifen, which we know is already effective in reducing the risk compared to no treatment. There has been a consistent 35–50% decrease in opposite breast cancers in the AI trials reported to date, giving strong clinical evidence that these agents may be superior to tamoxifen in breast cancer prevention.

The adjuvant trial results demonstrating a reduction in opposite breast cancers have led to the conduct of two primary prevention trials evaluating AIs in healthy postmenopausal women at increased risk for the development of breast cancer (Figure 3.3). The first of these studies is the National Cancer Institute of Canada Clinical Trials Group (NCIC-CTG) MAP-3 trial, a randomized double-blind, placebo-controlled study of the AI exemestane [77]. With a median follow-up of only 35 months, the exemestane-treated women had a 65% (0.19% vs. 0.55%; HR 0.35; 95% CI 0.18–0.70; $P=0.002$) reduction in the incidence of invasive breast cancer. There were numerically fewer ADH, ALH, LCIS, and DCIS in the exemestane group, but results did not reach statistical significance (0.16% vs. 0.24%; HR 0.65; $P=0.31$ for DCIS; 0.07% vs. 0.20%; HR 0.36; $P=0.08$ for ADH, ALH, or LCIS). A total of 4560 healthy postmenopausal women with increased risk entered the trial. Risk was determined based on a participant's being 60 years or older, prior breast biopsy showing atypical hyperplasia or LCIS, prior DCIS treated by mastectomy, or a Gail Model risk score of greater than 1.66% of developing invasive breast cancer over the next 5 years. The median age was 62.5 years, and the median Gail risk score was 2.3%. Adverse events of any grade were slightly more common with exemestane (88% vs. 85%; $P=0.003$), but the absolute differences between the groups for individual adverse events were small. Menopausal symptoms were frequent and more common with exemestane. The most frequent adverse events were hot flashes (40% vs. 32%; $P \leq 0.001$) and joint pain (30% vs. 27%; $P=0.04$). The use of AIs can reduce bone density and may result in bone fracture. In MAP-3, bone density measures were obtained at entry but not routinely during the trial. During treatment, reports of a diagnosis of osteoporosis were balanced in the two groups, and fracture rates were similar. The short median follow-up of the trial and patient selection (avoiding women with pre-existing osteoporosis) may be a factor in these initial results. With prolonged use of AIs, bone loss can be cumulative, and the development of osteoporosis in women who start AI therapy with a normal bone density is low, but for women who already have low bone mass, other breast cancer prevention options may be a better first choice.

Health-related and menopause-specific QOL was assessed using the MOS Short Form (SF-36) and the Menopause-Specific QOL questionnaire. There were no overall differences in the health-related QOL. Women receiving exemestane had an overall 7% worsening of menopause-related QOL compared to the placebo group.

Overall, the MAP-3 results are impressive and demonstrate that exemestane should be included with tamoxifen and raloxifene as an effective option for breast cancer prevention.

The second of these studies is the IBIS-II Trial, which will randomly assign 6000 post-menopausal women to receive either anastrozole or placebo. The primary endpoint of this study is the development of breast cancer. Other cancers, toxicities, cognition, and bone effects will also be evaluated. IBIS-II is being conducted in 40 centers in the United Kingdom and around the world.

Both IBIS-II and MAP-3 have placebo-control groups. While this design is scientifically compelling, a direct comparison with tamoxifen or raloxifene would allow a better risk/benefit evaluation. The IBIS-II study does have a separate component for DCIS patients that does compare anastrozole to tamoxifen and should allow some insight into the risk/benefit issue.

The NSABP has completed accrual to its 3000-patient B-35 study, which also evaluates tamoxifen and anastrozole in ER-positive DCIS. Ipsalateral and contralateral invasive and non-invasive breast cancers are the primary endpoints.

ASCO CLINICAL PRACTICE GUIDELINES (2009)

In 2009 the American Society of Clinical Oncology (ASCO) updated its Clinical Practice Guidelines on the use of pharmacologic interventions including tamoxifen, raloxifene, and AIs for breast cancer risk reduction [78]. As in the original 1999 guidelines and the 2002 update, these guidelines suggest that for women at increased risk for breast cancer, tamoxifen (20 mg/day for 5 years) may be offered to reduce the risk of invasive ER-positive breast cancer, with benefits for at least 10 years [79–80]. With the publication of the STAR results, the guidelines have been updated to state that for postmenopausal women, raloxifene (60 mg/day) may also be considered. A discussion of risk and benefits by health care providers is thought to be critical to patient decision making. The use of AIs and other potential chemoprevention agents is not now recommended outside of clinical trials.

PREVENTION OF ER-NEGATIVE BREAST CANCER

The benefits from SERMs in the risk reduction of breast cancer has been limited to preventing the development of ER-positive breast cancer. The results from treatment trials and the MAP-3 trial suggest that any benefits from AIs are also likely to be restricted to ER-positive tumors. Although ER-positive tumors represent the majority of breast cancers that occur, and these reductions represent a major advance, there has been substantial interest in identifying agents that could reduce the risk of ER-negative disease.

Retinoids are vitamin A derivatives and were best shown to have cancer preventative activity in patients with squamous cell carcinoma of the head and neck [81]. The synthetic retinoid fenretinide (N-4-hydroxyphenyl, 4HPR) has been evaluated in 2972 women with stage I breast cancer who were randomly assigned to receive either fenretinide 200 mg/day or placebo [82]. Overall, no benefit was demonstrated, but there was a suggestion of benefit in the reduction of both ipsalateral and contralateral breast cancer in premenopausal women. The benefit appeared to be independent of receptor status. A related follow-up study utilized a 2 x 2 design to evaluate low-dose tamoxifen (5 mg/day) and fenretinide in premenopausal high-risk women. The combination had favorable impacts on plasma insulin-like growth factor 1 (IGF-1) levels and mammographic density but did not reduce breast neoplastic events [83].

A variety of other agents, including retinoids, kinase inhibitors, statins, and COX-2 inhibitors, have been evaluated in the laboratory or in limited human studies. Outside current clinical trials, none of these agents are appropriate for risk-reduction therapy for ER-negative or ER-positive disease.

SUMMARY

The chemoprevention of breast cancer is in its infancy when compared to treatment and screening. The SERMs have demonstrated substantial clinical benefit in several large clinical trials, and one AI trial has also shown benefit, with others underway. The history of medicine has shown us that the greatest advances are often through the prevention of disease as opposed to its treatment. Although the current therapies have issues with side-effects, costs, and the identification of proper candidates for care, these are not insurmountable barriers. A report by Coopey and colleagues, entitled '*Clarifying the Risk of Breast Cancer in Women with Atypical Breast Lesions*' may represent a tipping point for breast cancer chemoprevention [84]. The authors identified 2942 women with atypical ductal or lobular hyperplasia, LCIS, or borderline DCIS/severe ADH seen at Massachusetts General Hospital, Brigham and Women's, and Newton Wellesley. The 10-year risk of invasive breast cancer for these women was 21.3%, but for those women who received chemoprevention the risk was reduced to 7.5%. This is the first large report of the use of breast cancer chemoprevention in routine clinical practice and is similar to the initial reports of statin use in patients who have dramatically elevated cholesterol levels. Preventive cardiology is now a routine component in all cardiology practices. The oncology community has always been supportive of cancer prevention strategies; chemoprevention represents a new opportunity to expand beyond lifestyle modifications.

Acknowledgements

The author thanks Barbara C. Good, PhD, for editorial assistance.

REFERENCES

1. Siegel R, Naishadham D, Jemal A. Cancer statistics, 2012. *CA Cancer J Clin* 2012; 62:10–29.
2. Hartmann LC, Sellers TA, Schaid DJ *et al.* Efficacy of bilateral prophylactic mastectomy in BRCA1 and BRCA2 gene mutation carriers. *J Natl Cancer Inst* 2001; 93:1633–1637.
3. Hartmann LC, Schaid DJ, Woods JE *et al.* Efficacy of bilateral prophylactic mastectomy in women with a family history of breast cancer. *New Eng J Med* 1999; 340:77–84.
4. Hong WK, Sporn MB. Recent advances in chemoprevention of cancer. *Science* 1997; 278:1073–1077.
5. Fisher B, Costantino JP, Wickerham DL *et al.* Tamoxifen for prevention of breast cancer: report of the National Surgical Adjuvant Breast and Bowel Project P-1 study. *J Natl Cancer Inst* 1998; 90:1371–1378.

6. Cuzick J, Forbes J, Edwards R *et al.* First results from the International Breast Cancer Intervention Study (IBIS-I): a randomized prevention trial. *Lancet* 2002; 360:817–824.
7. Cuzick J, Powles T, Veronesi U *et al.* Overview of the main outcomes in breast cancer prevention trials. *Lancet* 2003; 361:296–300.
8. Vogel VG, Costantino JP, Wickerham DL *et al.* Effects of tamoxifen vs. raloxifene on the risk of developing invasive breast cancer and other disease outcomes: the NSABP Study of Tamoxifen and Raloxifene (STAR) P-2 trial. *JAMA* 2006; 295:2727–2741.
9. Early Breast Cancer Trialists' Collaborative Group. Tamoxifen for early breast cancer: an overview of the randomised trials. *Lancet* 1998; 351:1451–1467.
10. Report from the Breast Cancer Trials Committee, Scottish Cancer Trials Office (MRC), Edinburgh. Adjuvant tamoxifen in the management of operable breast cancer: the Scottish Trial. *Lancet* 1987; 2:171–175.
11. Fisher B, Costantino J, Redmond C *et al.* A randomized clinical trial evaluating tamoxifen in the treatment of patients with node-negative breast cancer who have estrogen-receptor-positive tumors. *N Engl J Med* 1989; 320:479–484.
12. CRC Adjuvant Breast Trial Working Party. Cyclophosphamide and tamoxifen as adjuvant therapies in the management of breast cancer. *Br J Cancer* 1988; 57:604–607.
13. Rutqvist LE, Cedermark B, Glas U *et al.* Contralateral primary tumors in breast cancer patients in a randomized trial of adjuvant tamoxifen therapy. *J Natl Cancer Inst* 1991; 83:1299–1306.
14. Furr BJ, Patterson JS, Richardson DN *et al.* Tamoxifen (review). In: Goldberg ME (ed.) *Pharmacological and biochemical properties of drug substances*, Volume 2. Washington, DC: American Pharmaceutical Association, 1979, pp 355–399.
15. Adam HK. Pharmacokinetic studies with Nolvadex. *Rev Endocrine Related Cancer* 1981; (suppl 9):131–143.
16. Wakeling AE, Valcaccia B, Newboult E *et al.* Non-steroidal anti-estrogens-receptor binding and biological response in rat uterus, rat mammary carcinoma and human breast cancer cells. *J Steroid Biochem* 1984; 20:111–120.
17. Jordan VC, Fritz NF, Tormey DC. Long-term adjuvant therapy with tamoxifen: effects on sex hormone binding globulin and antithrombin III. *Cancer Res* 1987; 47:4517–4519.
18. Terenius L. Effect of anti-estrogens on initiation of mammary cancer in the female rat. *Eur J Cancer* 1971; 7:65–70.
19. Jordan VC. Effect of tamoxifen (ICI 46,474) on initiation and growth of DMBA-induced rat mammary carcinomata. *Eur J Cancer* 1976; 12:419–424.
20. Jordan VC, Allen KE. Evaluation of the antitumour activity of the non-steroidal anti-estrogen monohydroxytamoxifen in the DMBA-induced rat mammary carcinoma model. *Eur J Cancer* 1980; 16:239–251.
21. Wickerham DL, Fisher B, Wolmark N *et al.* Association of tamoxifen and uterine sarcoma. *J Clin Oncol* 2002; 20:2758–2760.
22. Abramson N, Costantino JP, Garber JE *et al.* Effect of factor V leiden and prothrombin G20210→A mutations on thromboembolic risk in the National Surgical Adjuvant Breast and Bowel Project cancer prevention trial. *J Natl Cancer Inst* 2006; 98:904–910.
23. Day R. Quality of life and tamoxifen in a breast cancer prevention trial: a summary of findings from the NSABP P-1 study. *Anna New York Academy of Sciences* 2001; 949:143–150.
24. Day R, Ganz PA, Costantino JP. Tamoxifen and depression: more evidence from the National Surgical Adjuvant Breast and Bowel Project's breast cancer prevention (P-1) randomized study. *J Natl Cancer Inst* 2001; 93:1615–1623.
25. King MC, Wieand S, Hale K *et al.* Tamoxifen and breast cancer incidence among women with inherited mutations in BRCA1 and BRCA2: National Surgical Adjuvant Breast and Bowel Project (NSABP P-1) breast cancer prevention trial. *JAMA* 2001; 286:2251–2256.
26. Narod SA, Brunet JS, Ghadirian P *et al.* Tamoxifen and risk of contralateral breast cancer in BRCA1 and BRCA2 mutation carriers: a case-control study. Hereditary Breast Cancer Clinical Study Group. *Lancet* 2000; 356:1876–1881.
27. Cuzick J, Forbes JF, Sestak I *et al.* Long-term results of tamoxifen prophylaxis for breast cancer – 96-month follow-up of the randomized IBIS-I trial. *J Natl Cancer Inst* 2007; 99:272–282.
28. Powles T, Eeles R, Ashley S *et al.* Interim analysis of the incidence of breast cancer in the Royal Marsden Hospital tamoxifen randomised chemoprevention trial. *Lancet* 1998; 352:98–101.

29. Powles TJ, Ashley S, Tidy A *et al.* Twenty-year follow-up of the Royal Marsden randomized, double-blinded tamoxifen breast cancer prevention trial. *J Natl Cancer Inst* 2007; 99:283–290.
30. Veronesi U, Maisonneuve P, Costa A *et al.* Prevention of breast cancer with tamoxifen: preliminary findings from the Italian randomised trial among hysterectomised women. Italian Tamoxifen Prevention Study. *Lancet* 1998; 352:93–97.
31. Veronesi U, Maisonneuve P, Rotmensz N *et al.* Italian randomized trial among women with hysterectomy: tamoxifen and hormone-dependent breast cancer in high-risk women. *J Natl Cancer Inst* 2003; 95:160–165.
32. Decensi A, Galli A, Veronesi U. HRT opposed to low-dose tamoxifen (HOT study): rationale and design. *Recent Results Cancer Res* 2003; 163:104–111 (Discussion 264–266).
33. Eli Lilly and Company. EVISTA (raloxifene hydrochloride): US prescribing information (online). Available at: http://pi.lilly.com/us/evista-pi.pdf (accessed February 24, 2012).
34. Hochner-Celnikier D. Pharmacokinetics of raloxifene and its clinical application. *Eur J Obstet Gynecol Reprod Biol* 1999; 85:23–29.
35. Escande A, Pillon A, Servant N *et al.* Evaluation of ligand selectivity using reporter cell lines stably expressing estrogen receptor alpha or beta. *Biochem Pharmacol* 2006; 71:1459–1469.
36. Sporn MB, Dowsett SA, Mershon J *et al.* Role of raloxifene in breast cancer prevention in postmenopausal women: clinical evidence and potential mechanisms of action. *Clin Ther* 2004; 26: 830–840.
37. Wolczynski S, Surazynski A, Swiatecka J *et al.* Estrogenic and antiestrogenic effects of raloxifene on collagen metabolism in breast cancer MCF-7 cells. *Gynecol Endocrinol* 2001; 15:225–235.
38. Glaeser M, Niederacher D, Djahansouzi S *et al.* Effects of the antiestrogens tamoxifen and raloxifene on the estrogen receptor transactivation machinery. *Anticancer Res* 2006; 26:735–744.
39. Anzano MA, Peer CW, Smith JM *et al.* Chemoprevention of mammary carcinogenesis in the rat: combined use of raloxifene and *9-cis*-retinoic acid. *J Natl Cancer Inst* 1996; 88:123–125.
40. Clemens JA, Bennett DR, Black LJ *et al.* Effects of a new antiestrogen, keoxifene (LY156758), on growth of carcinogen-induced mammary tumors and on LH and prolactin levels. *Life Sci* 1983; 32:2869–2875.
41. Osborne CK, Hobbs K, Clark GM. Effect of estrogens and antiestrogens on growth of human breast cancer cells in athymic nude mice. *Cancer Res* 1985; 45:584–590.
42. Balfour JA, Goa KL. Raloxifene. *Drugs Aging* 1998; 12:335–341 (Discussion 342).
43. Clemett D, Spencer CM. Raloxifene: a review of its use in postmenopausal osteoporosis. *Drugs* 2000; 60:379–411.
44. Johnston CC Jr, Bjarnason NH, Cohen FJ *et al.* Long-term effects of raloxifene on bone mineral density, bone turnover, and serum lipid levels in early postmenopausal women. *Arch Intern Med* 2000; 160:3444–3450.
45. Reid IR, Eastell R, Fogelman I *et al.* A comparison of the effects of raloxifene and conjugated equine estrogen on bone and lipids in healthy postmenopausal women: three-year data from 2 double-blind, randomized, placebo-controlled trials. *Arch Intern Med* 2004; 164:871–879.
46. Heaney RP, Draper MW. Raloxifene and estrogen: comparative bone-remodeling kinetics. *J Clin Endocrinol Metab* 1997; 82:3425–3429.
47. Ettinger B, Black DM, Mitlak BH *et al.* Reduction of vertebral fracture risk in postmenopausal women with osteoporosis treated with raloxifene: results from a 3-year randomized clinical trial. Multiple Outcomes of Raloxifene Evaluation (MORE) Investigators. *JAMA* 1999; 282:637–645.
48. Cummings SR, Eckert S, Krueger KA *et al.* The effect of raloxifene on risk of breast cancer in postmenopausal women: results from the MORE randomized trial. *JAMA* 1999; 281:2189–2197.
49. Cauley JA, Norton L, Lippman ME *et al.* Continued breast cancer risk reduction in postmenopausal women treated with raloxifene: 4-year results from the MORE trial. *Breast Cancer Res Treat* 2001; 65:125–134.
50. Burshell AL, Song J, Dowsett SA *et al.* Relationship between bone mass, invasive breast cancer incidence and raloxifene therapy in postmenopausal women with low bone mass or osteoporosis. *Curr Med Res Opin* 2008; 24:807–813.
51. Cummings SR, Duong T, Kenyon E *et al.* Serum estradiol level and risk of breast cancer during treatment with raloxifene. *JAMA* 2002; 287:216–220.
52. Martino S, Cauley JA, Barrett-Connor E *et al.* Continuing outcomes relevant to Evista: breast cancer incidence in postmenopausal osteoporotic women in a randomized trial of raloxifene. *J Natl Cancer Inst* 2004; 96:1751–1761.

53. Delmas PD, Bjarnason NH, Mitlak BH *et al.* Effects of raloxifene on bone mineral density, serum cholesterol concentrations, and uterine endometrium in postmenopausal women. *N Engl J Med* 1997; 337:1641–1647.
54. Barrett-Connor E, Grady D, Sashegyi A *et al.* Raloxifene cardiovascular events in osteoporotic postmenopausal women: four-year results from the MORE (Multiple Outcomes of Raloxifene Evaluation) randomized trial. *JAMA* 2002; 287:847–857.
55. Walsh BW, Kuller LH, Wild RA *et al.* Effects of raloxifene on serum lipids and coagulation factors in healthy postmenopausal women. *JAMA* 1998; 279:1445–1451.
56. Barrett-Connor E, Mosca L, Collins P *et al.* Effects of raloxifene on cardiovascular events and breast cancer in postmenopausal women. *N Engl J Med* 2006; 355:125–137.
57. Vogel VG, Costantino JP, Wickerham DL *et al.* Update of the National Surgical Adjuvant Breast and Bowel Project Study of Tamoxifen and Raloxifene (STAR) P-2 Trial: Preventing breast cancer. *Cancer Prev Res (Phila)* 2010; 3:696–706.
58. Stearns V, Johnson MD, Rae JM *et al.* Active tamoxifen metabolite plasma concentrations after coadministration of tamoxifen and the selective serotonin reuptake inhibitor paroxetine. *J Natl Cancer Inst* 2003; 95:1758–1764.
59. Desta Z, Ward BA, Soukhova NV *et al.* Comprehensive evaluation of tamoxifen sequential biotransformation by the human cytochrome P450 system in vitro: prominent roles for CYP3A and CYP2D6. *J Pharmacol Exp Ther* 2004; 310:1062–1075.
60. Jin Y, Desta Z, Stearns V *et al.* CYP2D6 genotype, antidepressant use, and tamoxifen metabolism during adjuvant breast cancer treatment. *J Natl Cancer Inst* 2005; 97:30–39.
61. Goetz MP, Schaid DJ, Wickerham DL *et al.* Evaluation of CYP2D6 and efficacy of tamoxifen and raloxifene in women treated for breast cancer chemoprevention: results from the NSABP P1 and P2 clinical trials. *Clin Cancer Res* 2011; 17:6944–6951.
62. Buzdar AU, Marcus C, Holmes F *et al.* Phase II evaluation of Ly156758 in metastatic breast cancer. *Oncology* 1998; 45:344–345.
63. Freedman AN, Yu B, Gail MH *et al.* Benefit/risk assessment for breast cancer chemoprevention with raloxifene or tamoxifen for women age 50 years or older. *J Clin Oncol* 2011; 29:2327–2333.
64. Land SR, Wickerham DL, Costantino JP *et al.* Patient-reported symptoms and quality of life during treatment with tamoxifen or raloxifene for breast cancer prevention: the NSABP Study of Tamoxifen and Raloxifene (STAR) P-2 trial. *JAMA* 2006; 295:2742–2751.
65. LaCroix AZ, Cummings SR, Delmas P *et al.* Effects of 5 years of treatment with lasofoxifene on incidence of breast cancer in older women. *Proc San Antonio Breast Cancer Symposium* December 11, 2008; Abstract 11: General Session 1, San Antonio, TX.
66. Goss PE, Strasser K. Aromatase inhibitors in the treatment and prevention of breast cancer. *J Clin Oncol* 2001; 19:881–894.
67. Nabholtz JM, Buzdar A, Pollak M *et al.* Anastrozole is superior to tamoxifen as first-line therapy for advanced breast cancer in postmenopausal women: results of a North American multicenter randomized trial. Arimedex Study Group. *J Clin Oncol* 2000; 18:3758–3767.
68. Bonneterre J, Buzdar A, Nabholtz JM *et al.* Anastrozole is superior to tamoxifen as first-line therapy in hormone receptor positive advanced breast carcinoma. *Cancer* 2001; 92:2247–2258.
69. Mouridsen H, Gershanovich M, Sun Y *et al.* Superior efficacy of letrozole versus tamoxifen as first-line therapy for postmenopausal women with advanced breast cancer: results of a phase III study of the International Letrozole Breast Cancer Group. *J Clin Oncol* 2001; 19:2596–2606.
70. Dirix L, Piccart MJ, Lohrisch C *et al.* Efficacy of and tolerance to exemestane (E) versus tamoxifen (T) in 1st line hormone therapy (HT) of postmenopausal metastatic breast cancer (MBC) patients (pts): a European Organization for the Research and Treatment of Cancer (EORTC Breast Group) phase II trial with Pharmacia and Upjohn. *Proc Am Soc Clin Oncol* 2001; 20:29a (Abstract 114).
71. Eiermann W, Paepke S, Appfelstaedt PJ *et al.* Preoperative treatment of postmenopausal breast cancer patients with letrozole: a randomized double-blind multicenter study. *Ann Oncol* 2001; 12:1527–1532.
72. Thüerlimann B. Adjuvant hormonal therapy for breast cancer: an evolving process (archived web conference). *Presented at Primary Therapy of Early Breast Cancer 9th International Conference* January 26–29, 2005; St. Gallen, Switzerland. Available at: www.medscape.com/viewprogram/3800_pnt (accessed February 24, 2012).
73. Jakesz R, on behalf of the ABCSG and the GABG. Benefits of switching postmenopausal women with hormone-sensitive early breast cancer to anastrozole after 2 years adjuvant tamoxifen: combined

results from 3123 women enrolled in the ABCSG Trial 8 and the ARNO 95 Trial. *Proc San Antonio Breast Cancer Symposium* December 8–11, 2004; San Antonio, TX.

74. Goss PE, Ingle JN, Martino S *et al.* A randomized trial of letrozole in postmenopausal women after five years of tamoxifen therapy for early-stage breast cancer. *N Engl J Med* 2003; 349:1793–1802.
75. Coombes RC, Hall E, Gibson LJ *et al.* A randomized trial of exemestane after two to three years of tamoxifen therapy in postmenopausal women with primary breast cancer. *N Eng J Med* 2004; 350: 1081–1092.
76. Baum M, Buzdar AU, Cuzick J *et al.* Anastrozole alone or in combination with tamoxifen versus tamoxifen alone for adjuvant treatment of postmenopausal women with early breast cancer: first results of the ATAC randomised trial. *Lancet* 2002; 359:2131–2139.
77. Goss PE, Ingle JN, Ales-Martinez JE *et al.* Exemestane for breast cancer prevention in postmenopausal women. *N Engl J Med* 2011; 364:2381–2391.
78. Visvanathan K, Chlebowski RT, Hurley P *et al.* American Society of Clinical Oncology clinical practice guideline update on the use of pharmacologic interventions including tamoxifen, raloxifene, and aromatase inhibition for breast cancer risk reduction. *J Clin Oncol* 2009; 27:3235–3258.
79. Chlebowski RT, Collyar DE, Somerfield MR *et al.* American Society of Clinical Oncology technology assessment on breast cancer risk reduction strategies: tamoxifen and raloxifene. *J Clin Oncol* 1999; 17:1939–1955.
80. Chlebowski RT, Col N, Winer EP *et al.* American Society of Clinical Oncology technology assessment of pharmacologic interventions for breast cancer risk reduction including tamoxifen, raloxifene, and aromatase inhibition. *J Clin Oncol* 2002; 20:3328–3343.
81. Hong WK, Lippman SM, Itri LM *et al.* Prevention of second primary tumors with isotretinoin in squamous-cell carcinoma of the head and neck. *N Engl J Med* 1990; 323:795–801.
82. Veronesi U, Mariani L, Decensi A *et al.* Fifteen-year results of a randomized phase III trial of fenretinide to prevent second breast cancer. *Ann Oncol* 2006; 17:1065–1071.
83. Decensi A, Robertson C, Guerrieri-Gonzaga A *et al.* Randomized double-blind 2 × 2 trial of low-dose tamoxifen and fenretinide for breast cancer prevention in high-risk premenopausal women. *J Clin Oncol* 2009; 27:3749–3756.
84. Coopey SB, Mazzola E, Buckley JM *et al.* Clarifying the risk of breast cancer in women with atypical breast lesions. *Proc San Antonio Breast Cancer Symposium* December 8, 2011; Abstr S4–4, San Antonio, TX.

4

Therapy of HER2 positive breast cancer

A. Bardia, J. Baselga

INTRODUCTION

Human epidermal growth factor receptors (HER) are potent activators of signal transduction pathways involved in cellular growth and proliferation. The HER family (also referred to as Erbb family) consists of four closely related type 1 transmembrane tyrosine kinase receptors: epidermal growth factor receptor (EGFR also known as HER1), HER2, HER3, and HER4 [1]. Each receptor consists of an extracellular domain with ligand binding property, a transmembrane lipophilic α-helical segment, and an intracellular domain with tyrosine kinase activity.

In the inactive state, HER exist as monomers with the extracellular domain in a tethered conformational state that prevents dimerization and subsequent receptor activation [2]. Binding of a ligand to the extracellular domain results in a conformational change exposing the β-hairpin arm of each domain to form pairs with other receptors [3, 4]. HER can form homodimers (two molecules of the same receptor) or heterodimers (two molecules of different receptors from the HER family) allowing for multiple receptor combinations [5]. The formation of the HER dimer then leads to activation of the tyrosine kinase domain and cross-phosphorylation of the tyrosine residues in the C-terminal tail segment [6]. The phosphorylation provides for docking sites for recruitment for a variety of signaling molecules that contain SH2 or PTB domains and results in the activation of intracellular signaling cascades, particularly the PI3K/AKT/mTOR and the RAS/RAF/ERK pathways, as depicted in Figure 4.1(a).

While structurally similar, each member of the HER family has unique properties. For example, in contrast with other HER family members, HER2 is a ligandless receptor and is constitutively in the conformation ready for dimerization. HER3 lacks innate kinase function, but is a potent inducer of heterodimer formation with other HER family members. While EGFR, HER2, and HER3 have been implicated in the pathogenesis and progression of various cancers, including breast cancer, the role of HER4 in oncogenesis is less clear.

ERBB2/HER2 ONCOGENE

HER2 is encoded by the *ERBB2/NEU/HER2* oncogene that drives malignant transformation, tumor proliferation, and metastasis [7, 8]. *ERBB2* gene amplification occurs in about 20–30% of human breast cancers, and HER2 overexpression is a significant and independent

Aditya Bardia, MD, MPH, Attending Physician, Massachusetts General Hospital Cancer Center, Boston, Massachusetts, USA.

José Baselga, MD, PhD, Physician-in-Chief, Memorial Sloan-Kettering Cancer Center, New York City, New York, USA.

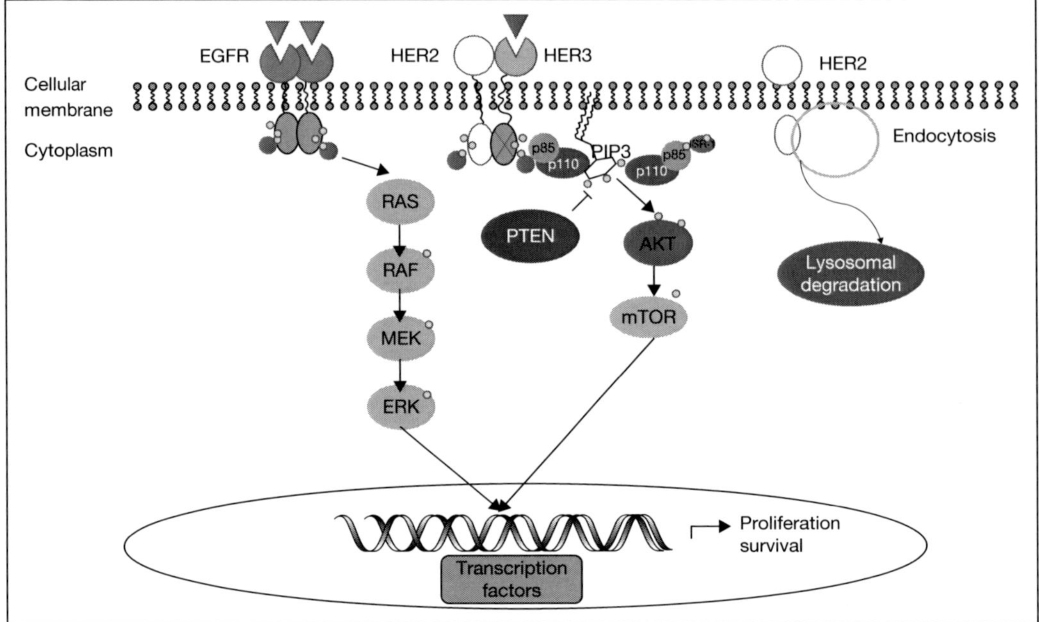

Figure 4.1(a) Schema outlining the HER2 signaling pathway and postulated site of action of major anti-HER2 therapies.

The formation of a HER dimer leads to activation of the tyrosine kinase domain and cross-phosphorylation of the tyrosine residues providing docking sites for recruitment for a variety of signaling molecules. The two principal intracellular signaling pathways of the HER family include the PI3K/AKT/mTOR pathway and the RAS/RAF/ERK pathway.

PI3K signaling is initiated when the p85 regulatory subunit of the PI3K alpha domain binds directly to the phosphotyrosine residues of the HER moiety. This leads to the phosphorylation of phosphatidylinositol 4,5-diphosphate (PIP2) to phosphatidylinositol 3,4,5-triphosphate (PIP3). PIP3 then sequentially activates phosphoinositide-dependent kinase 1 (PDK1) and AKT, which leads to phosphorylation of many other proteins, including mTOR (mammalian target of rapamycin), involved in cell survival.

ERK pathway signaling is initiated upon phosphorylation of RAS, a small GTPase, via tyrosine kinase activity. RAS in turns activates Raf which then activates mitogen-activated extracellular-signal regulated kinase (MEK1/2), and subsequently the downstream extracellular signal regulated kinase (ERK1/2). Once active, ERK1/2 phosphorylates a variety of proteins involved in cellular proliferation, differentiation and migration.

predictor of higher relapse and lower survival among patients with breast cancer [9, 10]. A truncated version of HER2, p95HER2, which lacks the extracellular domain but retains tyrosine kinase activity, is also frequently expressed in breast cancer [11].

ERBB2 amplification results in excess expression of the receptor on the cellular membrane facilitating formation of HER2 dimers. Although multiple homomeric and heteromeric dimer complexes can occur, the HER2–HER3 heterodimer is considered to be the most potent signaling pair, driving cell proliferation in HER2-positive cancers [12]. HER2 is also reported to induce EMT (epithelial-mesenchymal transition) changes in malignant cells that are critical for tumor invasiveness, migration, and self-renewal [13, 14].

HER2 over-expression may be an early event in the development of breast cancer since it occurs in up to 40% of ductal carcinoma *in situ* (DCIS), a higher frequency than in invasive breast cancer [15, 16]. HER2 over-expression also confers resistance to hormone therapy [17–19]. In the clinic, HER2 positive breast cancers show limited responsiveness to anti-

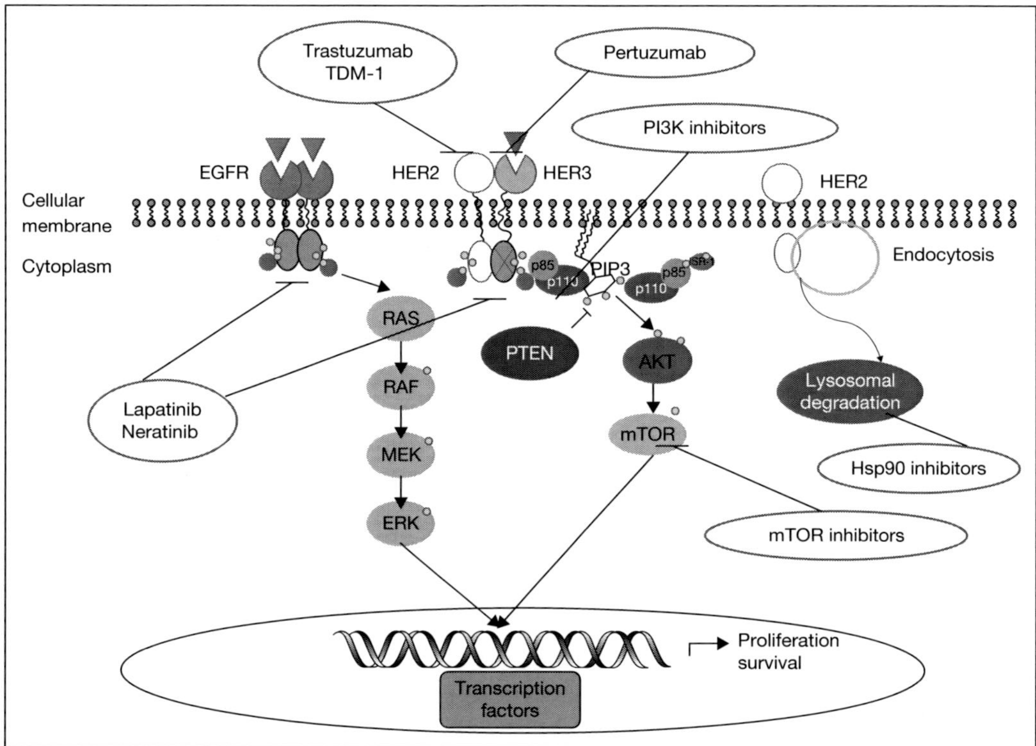

Figure 4.1(b) Schema outlining the postulated site of action of major anti-HER2 therapies in the HER2 signaling pathway.

Trastuzumab and TDM-1 bind to the extracellular domain IV of HER2, resulting in inhibition. Pertuzumab binds to the extracellular domain II of HER2 leading to inhibition of dimerization and subsequent activation of HER2. Lapatinib and neratinib inhibit the activity of the tyrosine kinase domain. PI3K and mTOR inhibitors inhibit downstream activation of the PI3K-Akt-mTOR pathway. Hsp90 inhibitors enhance ubiquitinylation and proteosomal degradation of HER2.

hormonal therapy [20, 21], and inhibition of the HER2 pathway improves patient outcome when combined with hormonal therapy [22, 23].

Taking into consideration the oncogenic role of HER2 in breast cancer, there is a strong rationale for targeting HER2 as a therapeutic approach in tumors with HER2 amplification. A number of approaches have been developed or are currently being evaluated. In this chapter, we will discuss therapies targeted towards HER2 inhibition in detail. We will review the rationale for drug development, the clinical development, and the current clinic status of individual therapy. The mechanism of action of the key anti-HER2 therapies is depicted in Figure 4.1(b) and the salient features are summarized in Table 4.1.

ANTI-HER2 THERAPIES

1. TRASTUZUMAB

Trastuzumab, a humanized monoclonal antibody, binds to the extracellular domain IV, close to the transmembrane domain, of HER2, leading to inhibition of the growth of tumors that over-express HER2 [24–26]. The tumor inhibition occurs via multiple mechanisms including:

Table 4.1 Salient features of drugs that inhibit HER2 pathway

Drug	Mechanism of action	Current clinical status
Monoclonal antibody		
Trastuzumab	Humanized monoclonal antibody that inhibits HER2	FDA approved for the first-line treatment of both localized and metastatic breast cancer
Tyrosine kinase inhibitor		
Lapatinib	Dual tyrosine kinase inhibitor of EGFR, and HER2	FDA approved for treatment of metastatic breast cancer
Neratinib	Second-generation, irreversible tyrosine kinase inhibitor of EGFR, HER2, and HER4	Ongoing phase II trials
Dimerization inhibitor		
Pertuzumab	Humanized monoclonal antibody that inhibits HER2 dimerization	FDA approved for treatment of metastatic breast cancer
Antibody drug conjugates		
T-DM1	Trastuzumab covalently bound via a thioether linker to DM1, a derivative of the potent antimicrotubule chemotherapy maytansanine	FDA approval for treatment of metastatic breast cancer is anticipated
Inhibition of PI3K/mTOR	Inhibits downstream PI3K signaling pathway activated by HER2	Ongoing phase III trials
Hsp90 inhibitor	Enhances ubiquitinylation and proteosomal degradation of HER2	Ongoing phase II trials
HER2 vaccine	Induces activation of peptide-specific cytotoxic T lymphocytes (CTLs) that recognize HER2 positive breast cancer cells	Ongoing phase II trials

FDA = US Food and Drug Administration.

- Inhibition of ligand-independent HER2 homodimerization [1]
- Prevention of proteolytic cleavage of the HER2 extracellular domain, resulting in lower levels of p95-HER2, the more active form of HER2 [27]
- Increased endocytotic degradation of the receptor [28]
- Increased antibody-dependent cellular cytotoxicity as the Fc portion of the human immunoglobulin G (IgG) segment of trastuzumab binds to immune effector cells [29]

Rationale for development

Soon after the identification of HER2, a number of groups developed murine monoclonal antibodies (mAbs) directed against the extracellular domain of HER and reported potent inhibition of HER2 over-expressing breast cancer cell lines [30–32]. However, theoretically, the efficacy of mAb4D5 in humans was limited by host immunogenic reaction against the anti-mouse antibody [33]. This led to the development of recombinant 'humanized' anti-HER2 monoclonal antibody, rhu-mAb HER2 (trastuzumab, Herceptin®), formed by combining the antigen binding loops from the murine antibody Ab4D5 with human variable region framework residues plus IgG1 constant domains [34]. In preparation for the clinical development of trastuzumab it was also demonstrated that the combination of anti-HER2 mAb with chemotherapy, such as doxorubicin, paclitaxel, and cisplatin, substantially enhanced antitumor activity over that of either agent alone [35, 36].

Clinical development

In the early 1990s, phase I and phase II clinical trials demonstrated that administration of trastuzumab was safe, well tolerated, and induced clinical responses. The initial single agent phase II study reported a clinical response rate of 12% in this heavily pretreated population ($n=46$) with HER2-positive metastatic breast cancer, thus representing the first demonstration of clinical activity with anti-HER2 therapy [37]. Importantly, no antibodies against trastuzumab were detected in patients, suggesting minimal host immunogenic reaction. A subsequent randomized phase III trial confirmed the efficacy of trastuzumab in combination with chemotherapy with improved objective response rate, disease-free survival (DFS), and overall survival in metastatic HER2-positive breast cancer [38]. This pivotal study was the basis for the regulatory approval of trastuzumab.

A number of subsequent studies have further clarified the activity of trastuzumab. Single agent trastuzumab, in a less pretreated population, is associated with a 20% response rate [39, 40]. The addition of chemotherapy, including paclitaxel, docetaxel, vinorelbine, capecitabine and cisplatin, further increases its clinical activity even among heavily pretreated patients [41–46]. Trastuzumab also increases the efficacy of hormonal therapy, although the clinical efficacy is less than with chemotherapy [22].

Trastuzumab is particularly effective in early breast cancer. Adjuvant trastuzumab use is associated with about 50% lower risk of breast cancer recurrence, as well as improvement in DFS and overall survival among women with localized HER2-positive breast cancers [47–51]. A comprehensive list of the randomized clinical trials evaluating trastuzumab therapy is provided in Table 4.2.

Current clinical status

Trastuzumab is currently approved by health authorities for the first-line treatment of both localized and metastatic HER2-positive breast cancer [52]. In the metastatic setting multiple chemotherapy combinations may be used, though trastuzumab with a taxane (paclitaxel or docetaxel) or with vinorelbine is usually preferred [53]. In the adjuvant setting, trastuzumab is universally recommended as a part of an adjuvant chemotherapy regimen for women with node-negative tumors with high-risk features, or node-positive tumors regardless of tumor size. The benefit of adjuvant trastuzumab for small node-negative tumors is unknown [54]. However, even small HER2-positive tumors carry a worse prognosis as compared to HER2-negative tumors [55].

The major serious adverse effect associated with trastuzumab is cardiotoxicity and adjuvant trastuzumab therapy is associated with a 1–4% risk of congestive heart failure [56]. While the exact mechanism of cardiac toxicity is unclear, a direct effect of HER2 blockade on cardiac myocytes appears to be the major culprit as in mouse models ventricular-restricted knockout of the *neu* oncogene results in the spontaneous development of dilated cardiomyopathy [57, 58]. Among the various chemotherapy regimen combinations, trastuzumab associated cardiotoxicity occurs with the highest frequency in combination with anthracyclines, possibly due to disruption of HER2 and heregulin by anthracyclines [59]. Elderly breast cancer patients with cardiac disease and/or diabetes are particularly at increased risk for cardiotoxicity and warrant more frequent monitoring [60].

Despite the major impact made by trastuzumab, many patients with HER2-positive metastatic breast cancer will experience disease progression due to primary or secondary resistance [61]. The major mechanisms for trastuzumab resistance include:

Table 4.2 Major randomized clinical trials evaluating efficacy of trastuzumab for HER2 positive breast cancer

Study	***Setting***	***Regimen***	***Sample size***	***Efficacy***
Slamon *et al.* [38]	Metastatic	Chemotherapy (doxorubicin or epirubicin plus cyclophosphamide, or paclitaxel), with or without trastuzumab	469	DFS: 7.4 vs. 4.6 months; *P* <0.001 OS: 25.1 vs. 20.3 months; *P*=0.01
Marty *et al.* [42]	Metastatic	Docetaxel, with or without trastuzumab	188	TTP: 11.7 vs. 6.1 months; *P*=0.0001 OS: 31.2 vs. 22.7 months; *P* = 0.0325
Gasparini *et al.* [43]	Metastatic	Paclitaxel, with or without trastuzumab	124	TTP: 369 vs. 272 days; *P*=0.030
Kaufman *et al.* [22]	Metastatic	Anastrozole, with or without trastuzumab	207	DFS: 4.8 vs. 2.4 months; *P*=0.0016
Joensuu *et al.* [47]	Adjuvant	Adjuvant docetaxel or vinorelbine, with or without trastuzumab	1010	DFS: 89% vs. 78%; HR 0.42; *P*=0.01
Piccart-Gebhart *et al.* [48]	Adjuvant	Adjuvant chemotherapy, with trastuzumab or without trastuzumab	1694	DFS: 85.8 vs. 77.4%; HR 0.54; *P* <0.0001
Romond *et al.* [49]	Adjuvant	Doxorubicin and cyclophosphamide (AC) followed by paclitaxel with or without trastuzumab	3676	DFS: 87.1% vs. 75.4%; HR 0.48; *P* <0.0001
Spielmann *et al.* [50]	Adjuvant	Anthracycline based chemotherapy with or without docetaxel, with or without trastuzumab	3010	DFS: 80.9% vs. 77.9%; HR 0.86; *P*=0.41
Slamon *et al.* [51]	Adjuvant	Doxorubicin and cyclophosphamide followed by docetaxel (AC-T), the same regimen trastuzumab (AC-TH), or docetaxel and carboplatin trastuzumab (TCH).	3222	DFS: 75% for AC-T, 84% for AC-TH, and 81% for TCH; HR 0.47; *P*=0.003 for AC-TH; HR 0.64; *P* = 0.06 for TCH

DFS=disease-free survival; HR= hazard ratio; OS= overall survival; TTP=time to progression.

- Impaired access of trastuzumab to HER2 extracellular domain due to truncated HER2 protein p95HER2 that lacks the extracellular domain but retains tyrosine kinase activity [62]
- Alternate signaling via other pathways such as IGF-1R (insulin growth factor-1 receptor) [63]
- Aberrant activation of downstream signaling due to PI3K mutations or PTEN loss [64]
- MUC1 (mucin 1, cell surface associated) [65]
- HER loss [66]

2. HER2 TYROSINE KINASE INHIBITORS (LAPATINIB, NERATINIB)

Rationale for development

Lapatinib (Tykerb®) is an oral, dual tyrosine kinase inhibitor that inhibits EGFR and HER2 signaling by reversibly binding to the ATP site, thus inhibiting receptor tyrosine autophosphorylation and subsequent activation of downstream signaling pathways [67]. Neratinib is an oral, irreversible, second-generation tyrosine kinase inhibitor that inhibits HER2 and is more potent than lapatinib [68].

In preclinical models, lapatinib was found to potently inhibit HER2 signaling and growth of HER2-positive cell lines and tumor xenografts [69, 70]. Although lapatinib is potent when given alone, the addition of lapatinib to trastuzumab markedly enhances its activity [70–72]. These observations provided a strong rationale to evaluate lapatinib in combination with trastuzumab in the clinic.

Clinical development

In early clinical trials, lapatinib was found to have clinical activity in heavily pretreated patients with HER2-positive metastatic cancers, including in patients with trastuzumab-resistant breast cancers [73]. A subsequent phase III trial comparing the combination of lapatinib and capecitabine, with capecitabine alone, among women with HER2-positive locally advanced or metastatic breast cancer ($n=324$), reported significant improvement in time to progression (8.4 vs. 4.4 months; $P<0.001$) with a hazard ratio (HR) of 0.49 [74]. While recent updated results failed to show an overall survival benefit (75.0 vs. 64.7 weeks; $P=0.21$), the study was underpowered for survival analysis, possibly due to high crossover (36%) following enrollment termination [75]. It has to be noted, however, that the initial first-line randomized trastuzumab study also had a high rate of crossover, and yet, an improvement in survival was observed [38]. Another large clinical trial evaluating the efficacy of the aromatase inhibitor letrozole in combination with lapatinib, versus placebo, among postmenopausal females with metastatic hormone receptor positive breast cancer ($n=1286$), reported significantly higher median progression-free survival with the lapatinib and letrozole combination, as compared to letrozole alone (8.2 vs. 3 months, HR 0.71; $P=0.02$) among women with HER2-positive tumors, but no difference among women with HER2-negative tumors [23].

As suggested by preclinical studies, the combination of lapatinib with trastuzumab is indeed superior, as compared to lapatinib alone. The clinical trial EGF104900 compared the activity of lapatinib alone or in combination with trastuzumab in patients with HER2-positive, trastuzumab-refractory metastatic breast cancer ($n=296$), and reported that the combination of lapatinib with trastuzumab was associated with improved progression-free survival (HR 0.73; $P=0.01$) and a trend towards improved survival (HR 0.75; $P=0.15$), as compared to lapatinib alone [76]. The NeoALTTO trial compared the efficacy of neoadjuvant therapy with lapatinib alone, trastuzumab alone, or lapatinib plus trastuzumab, for 6 weeks followed by paclitaxel for an additional 12 weeks among patients ($n = 450$) with localized, invasive HER2-positive breast cancer [77]. The pCR (pathologic complete response) rate was significantly higher with combined administration of lapatinib and trastuzumab (51.3%) as compared to trastuzumab (29.5%) or lapatinib (24.7%). Additional, smaller neoadjuvant studies have shown similar results [78–81].

Current clinical status

Lapatinib is currently FDA approved for (a) use in combination with capecitabine for treatment of patients with HER2-positive advanced or metastatic breast cancer who have received prior therapy including an anthracycline, a taxane, and trastuzumab; as well as (b) use in combination with letrozole therapy for postmenopausal women with hormone receptor positive, HER2-positive metastatic breast cancer as first-line therapy. However, it should be noted that lapatinib–letrozole combination therapy has not been directly compared to a trastuzumab based chemotherapy regimen for first-line therapy of HER2-positive metastatic breast cancer.

Like trastuzumab, the use of lapatinib in breast cancer is recommended for HER2-positive tumors only, as determined by either 3+ immunohistochemical staining (IHC) for HER2 protein, or *ERBB2* gene amplification (*ERBB2*/CEP 17 ratio >2) by fluorescence *in situ* hybridization (FISH). The most common clinical toxicity with lapatinib is diarrhea, which can occur in up to 60% of patients. Other adverse effects include hand-foot syndrome, nausea, rash and fatigue.

Unlike trastuzumab, lapatinib is active in women with brain metastasis due to its ability to cross the blood–brain barrier [82, 83]. Along the same lines, exploratory analysis of the lapatinib and capecitabine combination trial showed that patients in the lapatinib arm also had a lower incidence of brain metastasis than the capecitabine arm [74]. These findings were subsequently confirmed in a prospective clinical trial involving 242 women with progressive brain metastasis, wherein lapatinib was reported to reduce central nervous system (CNS) lesions in about 21% of patients with HER2-positive breast cancer [84].

Evaluation of lapatinib in the adjuvant setting, both as monotherapy and in combination with trastuzumab, is currently ongoing in multiple trials including ALTTO (NCT00490139) and TEACH (NCT 00374322). The ALTTO study is a large adjuvant study that has entered over 8000 patients and will definitively assess the role of lapatinib alone, and lapatinib in combination with trastuzumab, in early disease. If the study is positive it would lead to the registration of lapatinib therapy in early breast cancer. On the other hand, the TEACH study was designed to address a different question, namely if patients that had not received adjuvant trastuzumab would benefit from delayed administration of lapatinib. This study compared lapatinib versus placebo among 3161 patients that had been diagnosed with stage I–III HER2-positive breast cancer for a median of 2.7 years (range: 0.3–21.2 years) prior to study entry. The study failed to show a significant risk reduction with lapatinib [85]. Potential explanations for the lack of activity include the early relapse rate of HER2-positive breast cancer and the lack of central HER2-confirmation.

Neratinib has shown a robust response rate given as a single agent [86]. In a randomized clinical trial of women with HER2-positive metastatic or locally advanced breast cancer (n = 233), who received either neratinib monotherapy or the approved combination of lapatinib and capecitabine, a lower response rate with neratinib as compared to combination lapatinib and capecitabine therapy (29% vs. 40%) was observed [87]. It could be questioned whether this was an appropriate comparison given the presence of chemotherapy in the control arm. Interestingly, the combination of capecitabine and neratinib, despite the diarrhea that is induced by both agents, is doable and has shown a promising response rate [88]. Future details on the development plan of this very active agent are being awaited.

3. HER2 DIMERIZATION INHIBITORS (PERTUZUMAB)

Rationale for development

An important mechanism of HER2 signaling is via ligand-dependent HER2 activation. In particular, ligand binding to HER3 results in the formation of HER2:HER3 heterodimers, perhaps the most active HER2-containing heterodimer [12]. Trastuzumab does not prevent ligand-induced HER2 activation and therefore several approaches are being directed at interfering either with HER3 activation or with the formation of HER2:HER3 dimers [89].

Pertuzumab is a fully humanized monoclonal antibody that inhibits HER2 dimerization. Pertuzumab binds to HER2 receptor on the extracellular domain II, a different epitope on HER2 than trastuzumab (domain IV), sterically blocking receptor dimerization and subsequent downstream signaling [90].

In preclinical studies, combination of trastuzumab and pertuzumab had a synergistic antitumor effect in xenograft models when compared to either therapy alone [91–93]. The combination of trastuzumab and pertuzumab reduced levels of HER2 protein, blocked receptor signaling through Akt, enhanced antibody-dependent cellular cytotoxicity, and induced tumor regression in HER2-positive tumor xenografts.

The synergistic action of pertuzumab and trastuzumab may be explained by their complementary modes of action. Pertuzumab prevents the ligand-activated formation of HER2 heterodimers, while trastuzumab blocks ligand independent HER2 activation [89]. Furthermore, as the two antibodies are not competing for the same binding site on HER2 their combination may lead to a higher antibody load, thus eliciting a higher immune response and enhanced tumor inhibition via antibody-dependent cell-mediated cytotoxicity (ADCC).

Clinical development

Early clinical trials with pertuzumab given as single agent in non-HER2 over-expressing tumors showed disappointing results [94]. However, in a follow-up study of patients with trastuzumab-resistant HER2-positive breast cancer, pertuzumab in combination with trastuzumab had an overall response rate of 25% and clinical benefit rate of 50% [95]. These results led to a randomized clinical trial, CLEOPATRA (CLinical Evaluation Of Pertuzumab And TRAstuzumab) involving 808 patients with HER2-positive metastatic breast cancer who received placebo plus trastuzumab plus docetaxel (control group), or pertuzumab plus trastuzumab plus docetaxel (pertuzumab group) as first-line treatment. The pertuzumab group had significantly improved median progression-free survival (18.5 vs. 12.4 months, HR 0.62; $P < 0.001$), as compared to the control group, and a trend towards improvement in overall survival with pertuzumab based therapy [96]. The neoadjuvant trial, NeoSphere, also reported significantly higher pCR rates with combination of trastuzumab and pertuzumab with chemotherapy (45.8%), as compared to trastuzumab with chemotherapy (29%) or pertuzumab with chemotherapy (24%) [97]. Similarly, in the TRYPHAENA neoadjuvant trial, patients with localized HER2-positive early breast cancer were randomized to receive pertuzumab and trastuzumab either sequentially or concurrently with an anthracycline-containing or anthracycline-free standard regimen. Treatment with each regimen yielded similar but impressive pCR rates (45–66%, with no statistical difference between the arms), further confirming the potential benefits of dual HER2 blockade with pertuzumab and trastuzumab [98].

Current clinical status

Based on the results from the CLEOPATRA trial, it is anticipated that pertuzumab in combination with trastuzumab will be approved for treatment of metastatic breast cancer. Adverse effects possibly associated with pertuzumab therapy include diarrhea, febrile neutropenia, and dry skin [95]. Patients treated with pertuzumab did not have enhanced cardiac dysfunction as compared to trastuzumab [99]. A clinical trial evaluating the role of adjuvant pertuzumab and trastuzumab combination in localized early stage breast cancer, APHINITY (Adjuvant Pertuzumab and Herceptin IN Initial TherapY of Breast Cancer, NCT01358877), is ongoing.

4. HER2 ANTIBODY-DRUG CONJUGATES (T-DM1)

Rationale for development

Antibody-drug conjugates (ADCs) are mAbs to which highly potent cytotoxic agents have been attached, thus offering a mechanism of selectively delivering a cytotoxic load to tumor cells that express high levels of the targeted antigen. In humans, while HER2 is expressed in various tissues during fetal development, in adults the protein expression is low in normal epithelial tissues and only weakly detectable by IHC [100, 101]. Hence, this higher selective expression in tumors makes HER2 an ideal candidate to explore ADC-based approaches.

The key components of an ADC include the cytotoxic agent, a monoclonal antibody targeting a tumor-overexpressed or tumor-specific antigen, and a linker that covalently binds these components together. A prototype example for this class of agents in oncology is gemtuzumab ozogamicin, an anti-CD33 antibody linked to the cytotoxic antibiotic calicheamicin, developed for the treatment of CD33-positive acute myeloid leukemia [102].

Trastuzumab-DM1 (T-DM1) is an ADC comprising of trastuzumab covalently bound via a thioether linker to DM1, a derivative of the potent antimicrotubule chemotherapy maytansanine [103, 104]. The average drug-to-antibody ratio is approximately 3.5:1. T-DM1 uses trastuzumab to specifically localize HER2. Upon binding to the HER2, T-DM1 complex is internalized and degraded in lysosomes, releasing the active and highly potent chemotherapy (Lys-MCC-DM1) only to HER2 over-expressing cells [105]. In addition, T-DM1 retains the mechanistic properties of trastuzumab binding to HER2 to similar affinity as trastuzumab, and maintains the inhibitory properties of trastuzumab on HER2 signaling and ADCC [106].

A major issue in the clinical development of T-DM1 was the optimal choice of linker. In murine models, trastuzumab linked to DM1 through a non-reducible thioether linkage, displayed superior activity with minimal toxicity compared with unconjugated trastuzumab or trastuzumab linked to maytansinoids through disulfide linkers, and became the preferred linker choice for clinical development of T-DM1 [107].

Clinical development

In early phase I clinical studies, T-DM1 demonstrated encouraging anti-tumor activity with very limited toxicity among patients who had progressed on trastuzumab-based therapy [108]. In a follow-up phase II trial among patients with HER2-positive metastatic breast cancer ($n = 112$), who had tumor progression after being heavily pretreated with HER2-directed therapy and chemotherapy, an objective response rate of 25.9% was observed [109]. The toxicities were minimal with the most frequent grade ≥3 adverse events being hypokalemia (8.9%), thrombocytopenia (8.0%), and fatigue (4.5%). There was no dose-limiting cardiotoxicity. In another phase II trial, women with metastatic breast cancer ($n = 137$) were randomized to receive T-DM1 versus trastuzumab and docetaxel [110]. The response rate was slightly higher in the T-DM1 group (48%) compared with the trastuzumab–docetaxel group (41%), while the adverse events (grade >3) were significantly lower in the T-DM1 group (37.3%) compared with the trastuzumab–docetaxel group (75.0%).

The efficacy of T-DM1 was confirmed in the randomized clinical trial, EMILIA involving 991 patients with HER2-positive metastatic breast cancer who had previously been treated with trastuzumab and a taxane, received T-DM1 or lapatinib plus capecitabine. The T-DM1 group had significantly improved median progression-free survival (9.6 vs. 6.4 months, HR 0.65; P <0.001), as compared to the control group, and a improved overall survival in the T-DM1 group (30.9 vs. 25.1 months, HR 0.568 P <0.001) at interim analysis. T-DM1 demonstrated a benefit across all baseline characteristics, including ER/PR status, number of prior chemotherapy regimens, and presence of visceral metastases. The T-DM1 arm also had fewer side effects as compared to the lapatinib plus capecitabine arm [111].

Current clinical status

Based on the results from the EMILIA trial, it is anticipated that T-DM1 will be approved for treatment of metastatic breast cancer. Other large phase III trials evaluating the efficacy of T-DM1 are ongoing such as the MARIANNE trial (NCT00781612) evaluating T-DM1 versus trastuzumab and taxane, versus T-DM1 and pertuzumab, as the first-line therapy for metastatic HER2-positive breast cancer. Indeed, it is anticipated that T-DM1 could potentially substitute trastuzumab as the backbone of therapy in HER2-positive breast cancer and may be explored in combination with pertuzumab, potentially leading to a paradigm-shifting HER2 combination therapy free of conventional chemotherapy.

5. INHIBITORS OF DOWNSTREAM HER2 PATHWAY

(a) PI3K/mTOR inhibitors

Rationale for development

Mutations in the PIK3CA gene may be seen in about 25% of HER2-positive breast cancers [112], and the PI3K/AKT/mTOR pathway plays an important role in mediating trastuzumab response and resistance [64, 113–115]. Indeed, treatment of PTEN-deficient cells with PI3K inhibitors has been shown to restore trastuzumab sensitivity and inhibitory potential [116]. Retrospective biomarker studies have also suggested that tumors with constitutional activation of the PI3K-Akt pathway, such as PTEN loss and/or PIK3CA mutation, are resistant to trastuzumab [117–119]. Thus, combination therapeutic strategies utilizing PI3K or mTOR inhibitors along with trastuzumab could enhance the efficacy of trastuzumab and prevent emergence of resistance.

Clinical development and current clinical status

Prospective clinical trials combining PI3K and mTOR inhibitors with anti-HER2 therapies are currently underway. mTOR inhibitors are further ahead in the clinical development than PI3K inhibitors. In a phase II trial, the combination of the mTOR inhibitor everolimus and trastuzumab resulted in a clinical benefit rate of 34% with a median progression-free survival of 4.1 months among women ($n = 47$) with HER2-positive metastatic breast cancers that had previously progressed on trastuzumab-based therapy [120]. Results from the phase III trial, BOLERO-1 (Breast cancer trials of OraL EveROlimus-1, NCT00876395) and BOLERO-3 (NCT 01007942), investigating everolimus in combination with trastuzumab and chemotherapy (paclitaxel in BOLERO-1 and vinorelbine in BOLERO-3) as first-line treatment for metastatic HER2-positive breast cancer are eagerly awaited. Clinical trials evaluating anti-HER2 therapies in combination with PI3K inhibitors, such as XL-147, XL-765, GDC 0941, BKM120, are also underway (NCT01042925, NCT00928330, NCT01132664).

(b) Heat shock protein 90 inhibitors

Rationale for development

Heat shock protein 90 (Hsp90) is a molecular chaperone required for conformational maturation, stability, and activation of multiple mutated, chimeric, and over-expressed signaling proteins essential for the growth and survival of cancer cells [121]. Of the various oncogenic proteins, HER2 is one of the most important clients of Hsp90 [122], and Hsp90 inhibition enhances ubiquitinylation and proteosomal degradation of HER2 [123]. Furthermore, critical components of the HER2 signaling such as Akt are also client proteins of Hsp90 making it an attractive therapeutic target for HER2-positive breast cancer.

Geldanamycin, a benzoquinone ansamycin antibiotic, was one of the first Hsp90 inhibitors discovered [124]. Geldanamycin was found to selectively bind to the amino terminal ATP pocket of Hsp90 thereby preventing ATP binding and Hsp function. This led to the development of tanespimycin (17-allylamino-17-demethoxy-geldanamycin [17-AAG]), a geldanamycin derivative, as a potent Hsp90 inhibitor. Tanespimycin, particularly in combination with trastuzumab, was highly effective in inducing proteosomal degradation of HER2 and inhibiting tumor growth in breast cancer xenografts [125, 126]. Furthermore, tanespimycin was found to be effective against HER2-positive tumors with intrinsic resistance to trastuzumab, such as those expressing the truncated p95-HER2 [127].

Clinical development and current clinical status

Despite being an attractive therapeutic agent with exciting preclinical data, the clinical development of Hsp90 inhibitors has been difficult [128]. The initial clinical development of 17-AAG was limited due to its poor aqueous solubility and pharmacokinetic properties [129–131]. This led to the formulation of tanespimycin KOS-953 that contained polyethoxylated castor oil with better pharmacokinetic properties and was developed further clinically [132]. In a phase II trial, the combination of tanespimycin with trastuzumab reported a clinical benefit rate of 59% among patients ($n=31$) with HER2-positive metastatic breast cancer who had progressed on trastuzumab [133]. However, despite the impressive response rates, further clinical development of tanespimycin as an anti-cancer agent was suspended by the sponsor. Similarly, while IPI-504, alone and in combination with trastuzumab, was found to cause inhibition of tumor xenografts resistant to trastuzumab [134], the clinical development of IPI-504 in breast cancer has been suspended. Other Hsp90 inhibitors such as AUY922 are currently under clinical development (NCT01226732).

6. VACCINES

Rationale for development

Immunogenic peptides derived from oncogene product of *ERBB2* can induce peptide-specific cytotoxic T lymphocytes (CTLs) that recognize cancer cells expressing these peptides complexed with major histocompatibility complex class I molecules making this an attractive target for vaccine development [135]. Of the various immunogenic peptides, the most promising ones include E75, GP2, and AE37.

Clinical development and current clinical status

A major barrier to the development of cancer vaccines targeting tumor antigens has been immunologic tolerance. Based on murine model experiments, it was discovered that tolerance to Erbb2/Neu could be overcome by immunization to peptide fragments derived from the amino acid sequence of the intracellular domain or extracellular domain of rat Erbb2 protein, but not whole protein [136]. The immunogenicity of the peptide vaccine could be further enhanced with the use of immunoadjuvants such as granulocyte macrophage colony-stimulating factor (GM-CSF) that stimulate the mobilization of immunogenic dendritic cells to the site of antigen deposition [137]. These findings were subsequently confirmed in humans where the majority (92%) of patients developed T-cell immunity to HER2 peptides after receiving intradermal vaccination with putative $CD4^+$ T-helper epitopes derived from HLA-A2 binding motif of the HER2 protein and GM-CSF support [138].

As vaccines might work better when the tumor burden is relatively low, clinical trials have investigated HER2 vaccines in the adjuvant setting as a strategy to reduce risk of breast cancer. In a large clinical trial involving 168 women with high-risk breast cancer, E75 (HER2 369–377) with GM-CSF was given intradermally to previously treated, disease-free breast cancer patients [139]. As E75 binds primarily to HLA-A2 (40–50% of the general population), HLA-$A2^+$ patients were vaccinated, while HLA-$A2^-$ patients were observed prospectively for clinical recurrence (controls). It was reported that the vaccine was effective at stimulating HER2 specific immunity *in vivo*. The E75 vaccinated group had a significantly lower recurrence rate (5.6% vs. 14.2%; $P=0.04$) at a median of 20 months follow-up. However, the difference in recurrence decreased with further follow-up as the vaccine-specific immunity decreased over time suggesting the need for booster vaccinations. Reassuringly, toxicities were minimal with no significant difference between the treatment and control groups.

As trastuzumab enhances expression of the HER2 protein, combination immunotherapy with trastuzumab and HER2 peptide-based vaccines has been explored [140]. In a small clinical trial involving patients with metastatic HER2-positive breast cancer ($n = 22$), concurrent trastuzumab and HER2 vaccinations led to higher and longer immunity as compared to trastuzumab alone [141]. Similarly, the use of cyclophosphamide and doxorubicin chemotherapy has been reported to enhance tumor vaccine induced HER2-specific immunity among patients with metastatic breast cancer, suggesting that combination immunotherapy could be a promising therapeutic strategy [142].

While HER2 vaccine development is potentially promising, a number of barriers exist. First, while anti-HER2 vaccines can induce a specific immune response, the clinical benefits observed remain questionable. So far the clinical trials have been small and it has been difficult to evaluate meaningful endpoints. Second, vaccines carry the risk of development of auto-immunity [143]. Third, optimal dose, need for boosters, schedule, and duration of immunizations need to be defined well. Finally, careful assessment of toxicity is crucial as, unlike drugs, the side-effects of vaccines are less reversible and likely to persist for a prolonged period of time. A number of clinical trials testing HER2 vaccines as monotherapy, as well as combination with chemotherapy and anti-HER2 therapies, are currently ongoing, and should help address some of these issues (NCT0034109, NCT00095862, NCT00266110).

FUTURE DIRECTIONS IN DEVELOPMENT OF ANTI-HER2 THERAPIES

Looking into the future, we anticipate two major paradigm shifts in the field of HER2 targeted therapeutics: the increasing use of combinatorial anti-HER2 therapies, which possibly will pave the road to chemotherapy-free regimens, and the early use of neoadjuvant trials as the ideal testing ground in the development of anti-HER2 therapies. These concepts are discussed below:

1. COMBINATORIAL ANTI-HER2 THERAPIES

The management of HER2 breast cancer is rapidly moving towards combinatorial HER2 therapy, as shown by the success of trastuzumab in combination with lapatinib [76, 77] and trastuzumab in combination with pertuzumab [96, 97]. In both these studies the combination therapy was associated with significantly improved DFS. T-DM1 will likely be developed in combination with other anti-HER2 therapies and will offer the promise of developing a simple but highly active HER2 regimen free of conventional chemotherapy [144].

Combination therapies that have the potential of overcoming treatment resistance by inhibiting compensatory cross-talk between pathways will be particularly exciting. For example, while mutations in PIK3CA may confer resistance to lapatinib and trastuzumab, this can be restored through the use of PI3K/mTOR inhibitors, suggesting great utility of combination therapeutic strategies utilizing PIK3CA/mTOR inhibitors with lapatinib [145].

In order to develop effective and successful anti-HER2 combinations, predictive markers of response will need to be developed early in the translational trials to help identify distinctive features of each therapeutic agent. For example, breast tumors that express truncated HER2 (p95HER2) are resistant to trastuzumab, but may benefit from lapatinib therapy [62]. Similarly, increased expression of certain pre-treatment markers, such as p-Erk1/2, are important in predicting response to lapatinib [67]. Response rates to T-DM1 are higher among patients whose tumors express high median HER2 levels [109]. Such development of predictive biomarkers and identification of features unique to each therapeutic agent will facilitate smart combinations of HER2 therapies that could then be tested in neoadjuvant clinical trials as discussed below.

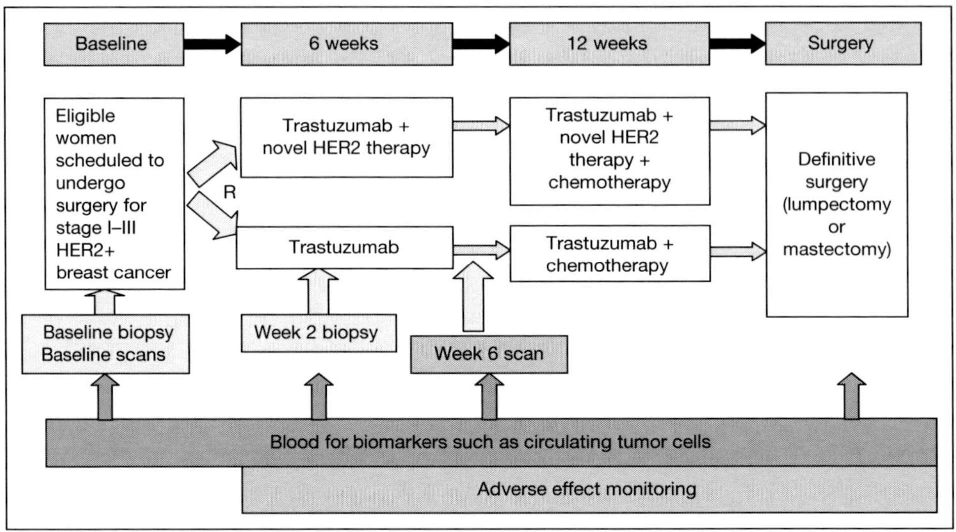

Figure 4.2 Schema of a neoadjuvant clinical trial design evaluating novel HER2 therapy.

In a randomized two-arm neoadjuvant study design, eligible women with biopsy-proven invasive breast cancer (T2 or higher), who are likely candidates for neoadjuvant trastuzumab therapy, are randomized to receive trastuzumab with the novel HER2 therapy (experimental arm), or trastuzumab only (control arm). A short lead-in phase with anti-HER2 therapy is built in to facilitate pharmacodynamic evaluation of the anti-HER2 therapy. After this 'biological window', patients continue on the same targeted therapy, plus standard chemotherapy such as weekly paclitaxel for 12 weeks, up to definitive surgery.

2. Neoadjuvant study design

Neoadjuvant administration of novel therapies offers the ability of *in vivo* assessment of response to a particular agent and the development of predictive biomarkers that can accurately predict response (or lack thereof) for an individual agent. While multiple combinations of HER2 therapies and permutations of study designs are possible, a randomized two-arm study design, similar to the NeoALTTO study design, is outlined in Figure 4.2, for the sake of simplicity. It should be noted that the primary endpoint of such a trial is difference in rate of pCR, a surrogate endpoint that has been shown to be a robust predictor of survival in HER2-positive breast cancers [146, 147].

Such a neoadjuvant study design has the potential to answer multiple questions rather quickly. For example, mid-treatment research biopsies similar to those used for early response to neoadjuvant endocrine therapies could be built in to identify early prediction of drug efficacy [148]. Non-invasive functional imaging modalities, such as PET (positron emission tomography) scans, could be incorporated for potential early prediction of efficacy [148]. Similarly, blood could be collected for serum biomarkers such as circulating tumor cells, which, if present, could facilitate interrogation of molecular changes and prognostic evaluation [150, 151]. Besides estimating pCR, paraffin slides could be analyzed for changes in various biomarkers such as downstream effectors of HER2 pathway such as p-AKT, p-ERK [66]. Thus, such a neoadjuvant study design can provide a huge repertoire for the successful development of biomarkers for personalized therapies. Indeed, the neoadjuvant approach has been shown to be successful in a number of neoadjuvant HER2 trials utilizing combinatorial HER2 therapies, as summarized in Table 4.3, and will likely replace traditional drug development in oncology.

Table 4.3 Neoadjuvant clinical trials evaluating combination of anti-HER2 therapies

Study	*Regimen*	*Sample size*	*Results*
NeoALLTO [77]	(A) Trastuzumab with paclitaxel weekly*12 (B) Lapatinib with paclitaxel weekly*12 (C) Trastuzumab and lapatinib with paclitaxel weekly*12	455	pCR 29.5% in arm A vs. 24.7% in arm B vs. 51.3% in Arm C *P*=0.32 B vs. A *P*=0.0001 C vs. A
GeparQuinto [78]	(A) Trastuzumab with epirubicin, cyclophosphamide (EC)*4 & docetaxel q3weeks*4 (B) Lapatinib with epirubicin, cyclophosphamide (EC)*4 & docetaxel q3weeks*4	620	pCR 31.3% in A vs. 21.7% in B *P* <0.05
TBCRC 006 [79]	Trastuzumab and lapatinib*12 (ER+ patients also received letrozole)		pCR Overall: 28% ER+: 21% ER–: 42%
Holmes *et al.* [80]	(A) Trastuzumab with FEC*3 then paclitaxel*12 (B) Lapatinib with FEC*3 then paclitaxel*12 (C) Trastuzumab and lapatinib with FEC*3 then paclitaxel*12		pCR in ER+: 40% in arm A vs. 21% in arm B vs. 58% in arm C pCR in ER–: 67% in arm A vs. 50% in arm B vs. 50% in arm C
CHER-LOB [81]	(A) Paclitaxel weekly*12, followed by 5-FU, epirubicin, cyclophosphamide (FEC) q3weeks*4 with trastuzumab (B) Paclitaxel weekly*12, followed by 5-FU, epirubicin, cyclophosphamide (FEC) q3weeks*4 with lapatinib (C) Paclitaxel weekly*12, followed by 5-FU, epirubicin, cyclophosphamide (FEC) q3weeks*4 with trastuzumab & lapatinib	121	pCR 28% in arm A vs. 32% in arm B vs. 48% in arm C *P* <0.05 C vs. A *P* <0.05 C vs. B
Neosphere [97]	(A) Trastuzumab with docetaxel q3weeks*4 (B) Pertuzumab with docetaxel q3weeks*4 (C) Trastuzumab and pertuzumab with docetaxel q3weeks*4 (D) Trastuzumab and pertuzumab q3weeks *4	417	pCR 29% in arm A vs. 24% in arm B vs. 45.8% in Arm C vs. 16.8% in arm D *P*=0.01 C vs. A *P*=0.03 C vs. B *P*=0.01 D vs. A

Table 4.3 Continued

Study	*Regimen*	*Sample size*	*Results*
TRYPHAENA [98]	(A) Pertuzumab and trastuzumab*6 with FEC*3 and then docetaxel*3 (B) Pertuzumab and trastuzumab*3 with FEC*3 (C) Pertuzumab, trastuzumab, docetaxel and carboplatin*6	225	pCR rates ranging from 45% to 66% with no significant difference between the arms
CALGB 40601 (NCT00770809)	(A) Paclitaxel weekly with trastuzumab*4 (B) Paclitaxel weekly with trastuzumab and lapatinib*4	400 (planned)	Clinical trial ongoing
TRIO/TORI B-07 (NCT00769470)	(A) Docetaxel, carboplatin, and trastuzumab (TCH)*6 (B) Docetaxel, trastuzumab, and lapatinib*6 (C) TCH and lapatinib*6	140 (planned)	
NSABP-41 (NCT00486668)	(A) Doxorubicin plus cyclophosphamide (AC)*4 followed by weekly paclitaxel with trastuzumab (B) Doxorubicin plus cyclophosphamide (AC)*4 followed by weekly paclitaxel with lapatinib (C) Doxorubicin plus cyclophosphamide (AC)*4 followed by weekly paclitaxel with trastuzumab and lapatinib	522 (planned)	Clinical trial ongoing

5-FU = fluorouracil; AC = doxorubicin and cyclophosphamide; EC = epirubicin and cyclophosphamide; ER = estrogen receptor; FEC = fluorouracil, epirubicin and cyclophosphamide; pCR = pathologic complete response.

The traditional drug model of taking drugs from phase I to phase II to phase III studies is slow, inefficient, and expensive with an estimated cost of $1 billion to $1.8 billion [152]. Furthermore, the early testing of new agents is done in heavily pretreated patients with metastatic cancer, which is not optimal as these tumors may have already evolved into a high resistance clone. It is not surprising then that traditional cancer drug development has had a high failure rate.

Use of a neoadjuvant model for drug development offers the promise of rapid and efficient triage of effective (and ineffective) drugs and the parallel development of biomarkers to guide patient selection for subsequent trials. Neoadjuvant trials should be conducted after efficacy of an agent is confirmed in phase I and II studies such as the use of pertuzumab in NeoSphere [97]. Results from the neoadjuvant trial would help determine the predictive biomarker(s) needed for selection of patients for future clinical trials, thus facilitating the development of smarter, smaller, and efficient clinical trials. The sample size, cost, and time required for completion of such a trial is much smaller than that of similar adjuvant studies, and can accelerate the successful development of the targeted therapy. For example, results from the NeoSphere trial [97] had suggested that trastuzumab and pertuzumab would be an effective combinatorial therapy for HER2-positive breast cancer almost a year before the results from the CLEOPATRA trial [96]. Such an approach represents a major paradigm shift from traditional drug development, but is desperately needed as the numbers of drugs, associated costs, and demand for personalized treatment regimens continues to accelerate.

SUMMARY

The development of the anti-HER2 antibody, trastuzumab, serves as a role model in oncology for successfully translating molecular discoveries into effective treatments. Indeed, neoadjuvant or adjuvant trastuzumab-containing regimens should be considered as the first-line therapy for all women with node negative (with high-risk features) or node positive HER2-positive breast cancer, as well as those with metastatic HER2-positive breast cancer. A list of commonly used trastuzumab-containing regimens is summarized in Table 4.4.

While many patients may ultimately progress on trastuzumab therapy, multiple strategies have been developed that can potentially delay or overcome trastuzumab resistance. This includes inhibition of HER2 dimerization (pertuzumab), inhibition of the tyrosine kinase activity (lapatinib), antibody-drug conjugates (TDM-1), inhibition of the downstream effectors of HER2 (such as PI3K/mTOR inhibitors) and enhanced degradation of HER2 receptors (Hsp90 inhibitors). Randomized phase III trials evaluating combination of trastuzumab with lapatinib, and trastuzumab with pertuzumab, have demonstrated remarkable success, and lapatinib and pertuzumab based regimens may be considered as second/third-line therapy after disease progression on trastuzumab (Table 4.4). Clinical evaluation of multiple other targeted therapies appears to be promising. Of note, even those patients that have failed prior regimens with trastuzumab, seem to continue to derive benefit from the continuous administration of trastuzumab.

In the years to come, practice-changing studies will include those investigating the role of lapatinib and pertuzumab in the adjuvant setting, the second- and first-line studies with T-DM1, and mTOR and PI3K inhibitors. It is also anticipated that there will be an increasing role for regimens with less chemotherapy or even chemotherapy-free combinations, representing a paradigm shift in the management of cancer.

Table 4.4 Commonly used anti-HER2 therapy based regimens

Regimen	*Dose and frequency*
	Adjuvant regimen
AC-TH[1]	Adriamycin/doxorubicin 60 mg/m^2 Cyclophosphamide 600 mg/m^2 every 3 weeks*four cycles, followed by Paclitaxel 80 mg/m^2 Trastuzumab 4 mg/kg loading dose and then 2 mg/kg weekly*12 weeks, followed by Trastuzumab alone, 2 mg/kg weekly or 6 mg/kg every 3 weeks, to complete a total 52 weeks of treatment.
ddAC-TH[1]	Adriamycin/doxorubicin 60 mg/m^2 Cyclophosphamide 600 mg/m^2 every 2 weeks*four cycles with pegfilgrastim, followed by Paclitaxel 80 mg/m^2 Trastuzumab 4 mg/kg loading dose and then 2 mg/kg weekly*12 weeks, followed by Trastuzumab alone, 2 mg/kg weekly or 6 mg/kg every 3 weeks, to complete a total 52 weeks of treatment.
TCH[1]	Trastuzumab 4 mg/kg loading dose and then 2 mg/kg weekly for 6 cycles concurrent with Docetaxel 75 mg/m^2 Carboplatin AUC 6 every 3 weeks*six cycles, followed by Trastuzumab alone 2 mg/kg weekly or 6 mg/kg every 3 weeks, to complete a total 52 weeks of treatment.
	Metastatic regimen
Paclitaxel and trastuzumab[3]	Paclitaxel 175 mg/m^2 every 3 weeks or 80 mg/m^2 weekly concurrent with Trastuzumab 4 mg/kg loading dose and then 2 mg/kg weekly or 8 mg/kg loading dose followed by 6 mg/kg every 3 weeks.
Docetaxel and trastuzumab[3]	Docetaxel 75–100 mg/m^2 every 3 weeks or 35 mg/m^2 weekly concurrent with Trastuzumab 4 mg/kg loading dose and then 2 mg/kg weekly or 8 mg/kg loading dose followed by 6 mg/kg every 3 weeks.
Vinorelbine and trastuzumab[3]	Vinorelbine 25 mg/m^2 weekly concurrent with Trastuzumab 4 mg/kg loading dose and then 2 mg/kg weekly or 8 mg/kg loading dose followed by 6 mg/kg every 3 weeks.
Lapatinib and capecitabine[4]	Lapatinib 1250 mg PO once daily on day 1–21 concurrent with Capecitabine 2000 mg/m^2 daily in two divided doses on days 1 to 14 every 21 days.
Lapatinib and trastuzumab[4]	Lapatinib 1000 mg PO once daily on day 1–21 concurrent with Trastuzumab 4 mg/kg loading dose and then 2 mg/kg weekly or 8 mg/kg loading dose followed by 6 mg/kg every 3 weeks.
Pertuzumab and trastuzumab	Trastuzumab 8 mg/kg loading dose followed by 6 mg/kg concurrent with Pertuzumab loading dose of 840 mg, followed by 420 mg concurrent with Docetaxel 75–100 mg/m^2 (at least six cycles) every 3 weeks.

[1] Can be used as first-line regimen. The efficacy of TCH is slightly lower than AC-TH suggesting that TCH should be preferentially considered only among certain patients such as those with contraindications to anthracyclines such as pre-existing cardiomyopathy.
[2] Can also be given as paclitaxel 175 mg/m^2 every 2 weeks with pegfilgrastim, or every 3 weeks.
[3] Can be used as first-line regimen.
[4] Can be used as second/third-line regimen after progression on trastuzumab based regimen.

REFERENCES

1. Yarden Y, Sliwkowski MX. Untangling the ErbB signaling network. *Nat Rev Mol Cell Biol* 2001; 2: 127–137.
2. Ferguson KM, Berger MB, Mendrola JM, Cho HS, Leahy DJ, Lemmon MA. EGF activates its receptor by removing interactions that autoinhibit ectodomain dimerization. *Mol Cell* 2003; 11:507–517.
3. Cho HS, Leahy DJ. Structure of the extracellular region of HER3 reveals an interdomain tether. *Science* 2002; 297:1330–1333.
4. Ogiso H, Ishitani R, Nureki O *et al.* Crystal structure of the complex of human epidermal growth factor and receptor extracellular domains. *Cell* 2002; 110:775–787.
5. Burgess AW, Cho HS, Eigenbrot C *et al.* An open-and-shut case? Recent insights into the activation of EGF/ErbB receptors. *Mol Cell* 2003; 12:541–552.
6. Ushiro H, Cohen S. Identification of phosphotyrosine as a product of epidermal growth factor-activated protein kinase in A-431 cell membranes. *J Biol Chem* 1980; 255:8363–8365.
7. Hudziak RM, Schlessinger J, Ullrich A. Increased expression of the putative growth factor receptor p185HER-2 causes transformation and tumorigenesis of NIH 3T3 cells. *Proc Natl Acad Sci USA* 1987; 84:7159–7163.
8. Di Fiore PP, Pierce JH, Kraus MH, Segatto O, King CR, Aaronson SA. erbB-2 is a potent oncogene when overexpressed in NIH/3T3 cells. *Science* 1987; 237:178–182.
9. Slamon DJ, Clark GM, Wong SG *et al.* Human breast cancer: correlation of relapse and survival with amplification of the HER-2/neu oncogene. *Science* 1987; 235:177–182.
10. Tandon AK, Clark GM, Chamness GC, Ullrich A, McGuire WL. HER-2/neu oncogene protein and prognosis in breast cancer. *J Clin Oncol* 1989; 7:1120–1128.
11. Arribas J, Baselga J, Pedersen K, Parra-Palau JL. p95HER-2 and breast cancer. *Cancer Res* 2011; 71: 1515–1519 (review).
12. Klapper LN, Glathe S, Vaisman N *et al.* The ErbB-2/HER-2 oncoprotein of human carcinomas may function solely as a shared coreceptor for multiple stroma-derived growth factors. *Proc Natl Acad Sci USA* 1999; 96:4995–5000.
13. Kim IY, Yong HY, Kang KW, Moon A. Overexpression of ErbB2 induces invasion of MCF10A human breast epithelial cells via MMP-9. *Cancer Lett* 2009; 275:227–233.
14. Weinberg RA. Twisted epithelial-mesenchymal transition blocks senescence. *Nat Cell Biol* 2008; 10:1021–1023.
15. Tamimi RM, Baer HJ, Marotti J *et al.* Comparison of molecular phenotypes of ductal carcinoma in situ and invasive breast cancer. *Breast Cancer Res* 2008; 10:R67 [Epub 2008 Aug 5].
16. Clark SE, Warwick J, Carpenter R, Bowen RL, Duffy SW, Jones JL. Molecular subtyping of DCIS: heterogeneity of breast cancer reflected in pre-invasive disease. *Br J Cancer* 2011; 104:120–127.
17. Benz CC, Scott GK, Sarup JC *et al.* Estrogen-dependent, tamoxifen-resistant tumorigenic growth of MCF-7 cells transfected with HER-2/neu. *Breast Cancer Res Treat* 1992; 24:85–95.
18. De Laurentiis M. Arpino G, Massarelli E *et al.* A meta-analysis on the interaction between HER-2 expression and response to endocrine treatment in advanced breast cancer. *Clin Cancer Res* 2005; 11:4741–4748.
19. Shou J, Massarweh S, Osborne CK *et al.* Mechanisms of tamoxifen resistance: increased estrogen receptor-HER-2/neu cross-talk in ER/HER-2-positive breast cancer. *J Natl Cancer Inst* 2004; 96:926–935.
20. Dowsett M, Houghton J, Iden C *et al.* Benefit from adjuvant tamoxifen therapy in primary breast cancer patients according oestrogen receptor, progesterone receptor, EGF receptor and HER-2 status. *Ann Oncol* 2006; 17:818–826.
21. Linderholm B, Bergqvist J, Hellborg H *et al.* Shorter survival-times following adjuvant endocrine therapy in oestrogen- and progesterone-receptor positive breast cancer overexpressing HER2 and/or with an increased expression of vascular endothelial growth factor. *Med Oncol* 2009; 26:480–490.
22. Kaufman B, Mackey JR, Clemens MR *et al.* Trastuzumab plus anastrozole versus anastrozole alone for the treatment of postmenopausal women with human epidermal growth factor receptor 2-positive, hormone-receptor-positive metastatic breast cancer: results from the randomized phase III TAnDEM study. *J Clin Oncol* 2009; 27:5529–5537.
23. Johnston S, Pippen J Jr, Pivot X *et al.* Lapatinib combined with letrozole vs letrozole and placebo as first-line therapy for postmenopausal hormone receptor-positive metastatic breast cancer. *J Clin Oncol* 2009; 27:5538–5546.

24. Cho HS, Mason K, Ramyar KX *et al.* Structure of the extracellular region of HER-2 alone and in complex with the Herceptin Fab. *Nature* 2003; 421:756–760.
25. Tokuda Y, Ohnishi Y, Shimamura K *et al.* In vitro and in vivo anti-tumour effects of a humanised monoclonal antibody against c-erbB-2 product. *Br J Cancer* 1996; 73:1362–1365.
26. Mariani G, Fasolo A, De Benedictis E, Gianni L. Trastuzumab as adjuvant systemic therapy for HER-2-positive breast cancer. *Nat Clin Pract Oncol* 2009; 6:93–104.
27. Molina MA, Codony-Servat J, Albanell J, Rojo F, Arribas J, Baselga J. Trastuzumab (herceptin), a humanized anti-HER-2 receptor monoclonal antibody, inhibits basal and activated HER-2 ectodomain cleavage in breast cancer cells. *Cancer Res* 2001; 61:4744–4749.
28. Spector NL, Blackwell KL. Understanding the mechanisms behind trastuzumab therapy for human epidermal growth factor receptor 2-positive breast cancer. *J Clin Oncol* 2009; 27:5838–5847 (review).
29. Clynes RA, Towers TL, Presta LG, Ravetch JV. Inhibitory Fc receptors modulate in vivo cytotoxicity against tumor targets. *Nat Med* 2000; 6:443–446.
30. Drebin JA, Stern DF, Link VC, Weinberg RA, Greene MI. Monoclonal antibodies identify a cell-surface antigen associated with an activated cellular oncogene. *Nature* 1984; 312:545–548.
31. Hudziak RM, Lewis GD, Winget M, Fendly BM, Shepard HM, Ullrich A. p185HER-2 monoclonal antibody has antiproliferative effects in vitro and sensitizes human breast tumor cells to tumor necrosis factor. *Mol Cell Biol* 1989; 9:1165–1172.
32. Lewis GD, Figari I, Fendly B *et al.* Differential responses of human tumor cell lines to anti-pl85HER-2 monoclonal antibodies. *Cancer Immunol Immunother* 1993; 37:255–263.
33. Shepard HM, Lewis GD, Sarup JC *et al.* Monoclonal antibody therapy of human cancer: taking the HER-2 protooncogene to the clinic. *J Clin Immunol* 1991; 11:117–127 (review).
34. Carter P, Presta L, Gorman CM *et al.* Humanization of an anti-p185HER2 antibody for human cancer therapy. *Proc Natl Acad Sci USA* 1992; 89:4285–4289.
35. Baselga J, Norton L, Albanell J, Kim YM, Mendelsohn J. Recombinant humanized anti-HER-2 antibody (Herceptin) enhances the antitumor activity of paclitaxel and doxorubicin against HER-2 /neu overexpressing human breast cancer xenografts. *Cancer Res* 1998; 58:2825–2831.
36. Pietras RJ, Fendly BM, Chazin VR, Pegram MD, Howell SB, Slamon DJ. Antibody to HER-2/neu receptor blocks DNA repair after cisplatin in human breast and ovarian cancer cells. *Oncogene* 1994; 9:1829–1838.
37. Baselga J, Tripathy D, Mendelsohn J *et al.* Phase II study of weekly intravenous recombinant humanized anti-pl85HER-2 monoclonal antibody in patients with HER-2/neu-overexpressing metastatic breast cancer. *J Clin Oncol* 1996; 14:737–744.
38. Slamon DJ, Leyland-Jones B, Shak S *et al.* Use of chemotherapy plus a monoclonal antibody against HER-2 for metastatic breast cancer that overexpresses HER-2. *N Engl J Med* 2001; 344:783–792.
39. Cobleigh MA, Vogel CL, Tripathy D *et al.* Multinational study of the efficacy and safety of humanized anti-HER2 monoclonal antibody in women who have HER2-overexpressing metastatic breast cancer that has progressed after chemotherapy for metastatic disease. *J Clin Oncol* 1999; 17:2639–2648.
40. Baselga J, Carbonell X, Castañeda-Soto NJ *et al.* Phase II study of efficacy, safety, and pharmacokinetics of trastuzumab monotherapy administered on a 3-weekly schedule. *J Clin Oncol* 2005; 23:2162–2171.
41. Andersson M, Lidbrink E, Bjerre K *et al.* Phase III randomized study comparing docetaxel plus trastuzumab with vinorelbine plus trastuzumab as first-line therapy of metastatic or locally advanced human epidermal growth factor receptor 2-positive breast cancer: the HERNATA study. *J Clin Oncol* 2011; 29:264–271.
42. Marty M, Cognetti F, Maraninchi D *et al.* Randomized phase II trial of the efficacy and safety of trastuzumab combined with docetaxel in patients with human epidermal growth factor receptor 2-positive metastatic breast cancer administered as first-line treatment: the M77001 study group. *J Clin Oncol* 2005; 23:4265–4274.
43. Gasparini G, Gion M, Mariani L *et al.* Randomized phase II trial of weekly paclitaxel alone versus trastuzumab plus weekly paclitaxel as first-line therapy of patients with Her-2 positive advanced breast cancer. *Breast Cancer Res Treat* 2007; 101:355–365.
44. von Minckwitz G, Schwedler K, Schmidt M *et al.* GBG 26/BIG 03–05 study group and participating investigators. Trastuzumab beyond progression: overall survival analysis of the GBG 26/BIG 3–05 phase III study in HER-2-positive breast cancer. *Eur J Cancer* 2011; 47:2273–2281.
45. Bartsch R, Wenzel C, Altorjai G *et al.* Capecitabine and trastuzumab in heavily pretreated metastatic breast cancer. *J Clin Oncol* 2007; 25:3853–3858.

46. Harris CA, Ward RL, Dobbins TA, Drew AK, Pearson S. The efficacy of HER2-targeted agents in metastatic breast cancer: a meta-analysis. *Ann Oncol* 2011; 22:1308–1317.
47. Joensuu H, Kellokumpu-Lehtinen PL, Bono P *et al*. Adjuvant docetaxel or vinorelbine with or without trastuzumab for breast cancer. *N Engl J Med* 2006; 354:809–820.
48. Piccart-Gebhart MJ, Procter M, Leyland-Jones B *et al*. Trastuzumab after adjuvant chemotherapy in HER2-positive breast cancer. *N Engl J Med* 2005; 353:1659–1672.
49. Romond EH, Perez EA, Bryant J *et al*. Trastuzumab plus adjuvant chemotherapy for operable HER2-positive breast cancer. *N Engl J Med* 2005; 353:1673–1684.
50. Spielmann M, Roché H, Delozier T *et al*. Trastuzumab for patients with axillary-node-positive breast cancer: results of the FNCLCC-PACS 04 trial. *J Clin Oncol* 2009; 27:6129–6134.
51. Slamon D, Eiermann W, Robert N *et al*. Breast Cancer International Research Group. Adjuvant trastuzumab in HER2-positive breast cancer. *N Engl J Med* 2011; 365:1273–1283.
52. Hudis CA. Trastuzumab – mechanism of action and use in clinical practice. *N Engl J Med* 2007; 357: 39–51 (review).
53. Lin NU, Winer EP. Chemotherapy agents in human epidermal growth factor receptor 2-positive breast cancer: time to step out of the limelight. *J Clin Oncol* 2011; 29:251–253.
54. Banerjee S, Smith IE. Management of small HER-2-positive breast cancers. *Lancet Oncol* 2010; 11: 1193–1199 (review).
55. Gonzalez-Angulo AM, Litton JK, Broglio KR *et al*. High risk of recurrence for patients with breast cancer who have human epidermal growth factor receptor 2-positive, node-negative tumors 1 cm or smaller. *J Clin Oncol* 2009; 27:5700–5706.
56. Russell SD, Blackwell KL, Lawrence J *et al*. Independent adjudication of symptomatic heart failure with the use of doxorubicin and cyclophosphamide followed by trastuzumab adjuvant therapy: a combined review of cardiac data from the National Surgical Adjuvant breast and Bowel Project B-31 and the North Central Cancer Treatment Group N9831 clinical trials. *J Clin Oncol* 2010; 28:3416–3421.
57. Crone SA, Zhao YY, Fan L *et al*. ERB2 is essential in the prevention of dilated cardiomyopathy. *Nat Med* 2002; 8:459–465.
58. de Azambuja E, Bedard PL, Suter T *et al*. Cardiac toxicity with anti-HER-2 therapies: what have we learned so far? *Target Oncol* 2009; 4:77–88.
59. de Korte MA, de Vries EG, Lub-de Hooge MN *et al*. 111 Indium-trastuzumab visualises myocardial human epidermal growth factor receptor 2 expression shortly after anthracycline treatment but not during heart failure: a clue to uncover the mechanisms of trastuzumab-related cardiotoxicity. *Eur J Cancer* 2007; 43:2046–2051.
60. Serrano C, Cortés J, De Mattos-Arruda L *et al*. Trastuzumab-related cardiotoxicity in the elderly: a role for cardiovascular risk factors. *Ann Oncol* 2011; Aug 9 [Epub ahead of print].
61. Nahta R, Esteva FJ. Herceptin: mechanisms of action and resistance. *Cancer Lett* 2006; 232:123–138.
62. Scaltriti M, Rojo F, Ocaña A *et al*. Expression of p95HER-2, a truncated form of the HER-2 receptor, and response to anti-HER-2 therapies in breast cancer. *J Natl Cancer Inst* 2007; 99:628–638.
63. Lu Y, Zi X, Zhao Y, Mascarenhas D, Pollak M. Insulin-like growth factor-I receptor signaling and resistance to trastuzumab (Herceptin). *J Natl Cancer Inst* 2001; 93:1852–1857.
64. Berns K, Horlings HM, Hennessy BT *et al*. A functional genetic approach identifies the PI3K pathway as a major determinant of trastuzumab resistance in breast cancer. *Cancer Cell* 2007; 12:395–402.
65. Fessler SP, Wotkowicz MT, Mahanta SK, Bamdad C. MUC1* is a determinant of trastuzumab (Herceptin) resistance in breast cancer cells. *Breast Cancer Res Treat* 2009; 118:113–124.
66. Mittendorf EA, Wu Y, Scaltriti M *et al*. Loss of HER-2 amplification following trastuzumab-based neoadjuvant systemic therapy and survival outcomes. *Clin Cancer Res* 2009; 15:7381–7388.
67. Spector NL, Xia W, Burris H III *et al*. Study of the biological effects of lapatinib, a reversible inhibitor of ErbB1 and ErbB2 tyrosine kinases, on tumor growth and survival pathways in patients with advanced malignancies. *J Clin Oncol* 2005; 23:2502–2512.
68. Rabindran SK, Discafani, Rosflord EC *et al*. Anti-tumor activity of HKI-272, an orally active, irreversible inhibitor of the HER-2 tyrosine kinase. *Cancer Res* 2004; 64:3958–3965.
69. Konecny GE, Pegram MD, Venkatesan N *et al*. Activity of the dual kinase inhibitor lapatinib (GW572016) against HER-2-overexpressing and trastuzumab-treated breast cancer cells. *Cancer Res* 2006; 66:1630–1639.

70. Scaltriti M, Verma C, Guzman M *et al*. Lapatinib, a HER2 tyrosine kinase inhibitor, induces stabilization and accumulation of HER2 and potentiates trastuzumab-dependent cell cytotoxicity. *Oncogene* 2009; 28:803–814.
71. Xia W, Gerard CM, Liu L, Baudson NM, Ory TL, Spector NL. Combining lapatinib (GW572016), a small molecule inhibitor of ErbB1 and ErbB2 tyrosine kinases, with therapeutic anti-ErbB2 antibodies enhances apoptosis of ErbB2-overexpressing breast cancer cells. *Oncogene* 2005; 24:6213–6221.
72. Rimawi MF, Wiechmann LS, Wang YC *et al*. Reduced dose and intermittent treatment with lapatinib and trastuzumab for potent blockade of the HER pathway in HER2/neu-overexpressing breast tumor xenografts. *Clin Cancer Res* 2011; 17:1351–1361.
73. Burris HA III. Dual kinase inhibition in the treatment of breast cancer: initial experience with the EGFR/ErbB-2 inhibitor lapatinib. *Oncologist* 2004; 9:10–15 (review).
74. Geyer CE, Forster J, Lindquist D *et al*. Lapatinib plus capecitabine for HER-2-positive advanced breast cancer. *N Engl J Med* 2006; 355:2733–2743.
75. Cameron D, Casey M, Oliva C, Newstat B, Imwalle B, Geyer CE. Lapatinib plus capecitabine in women with HER-2-positive advanced breast cancer: final survival analysis of a phase III randomized trial. *Oncologist* 2010; 15:924–934.
76. Blackwell KL, Burstein HJ, Storniolo AM *et al*. Randomized study of lapatinib alone or in combination with trastuzumab in women with ErbB2-positive, trastuzumab-refractory metastatic breast cancer. *J Clin Oncol* 2010; 28:1124–1130.
77. Baselga J, Bradbury I, Eidtmann H *et al*. Lapatinib with trastuzumab for HER2-positive early breast cancer (NeoALTTO): a randomised, open-label, multicentre, phase 3 trial. *Lancet* 2012; 379:633–640.
78. Untch M, Loibl S, Bischoff J *et al*. Lapatinib versus trastuzumab in combination with neoadjuvant anthracycline-taxane-based chemotherapy (GeparQuinto, GBG 44): a randomised phase 3 trial. *Lancet Oncology* 2012; 13:135–144 [Epub 2012 Jan 17].
79. Chang JC, Mayer IA, Forero-Torres A *et al*. On behalf of the Translational Breast Cancer Research Consortium. TBCRC 006: a multicenter phase II study of neoadjuvant lapatinib and trastuzumab in patients with HER2-overexpressing breast cancer. *J Clin Oncol* 2011; 29(suppl):Abstract 505.
80. Holmes FA, Espina V, Liotta LA *et al*. Correlation of clinical and molecular findings with pathologic response to preoperative lapatinib and trastuzumab, separately or in combination, prior to neoadjuvant chemotherapy for HER2 positive breast cancer. Abstract # S5-7. Presented at San Antonio Breast Cancer Conference, San Antonio (USA), 2011.
81. Guarneri V, Frassoldati A, Bottini A *et al*. Final results of a phase II randomized trial of neoadjuvant anthracycline-taxane chemotherapy plus lapatinib, trastuzumab, or both in HER-2-positive breast cancer (CHER-LOB trial). *J Clin Oncol* 2011; 29(suppl):Abstract 507.
82. Lin NU, Bellon JR, Winer EP. CNS metastases in breast cancer. *J Clin Oncol* 2004; 22:3608–3617.
83. Gril B, Palmieri D, Bronder JL *et al*. Effect of lapatinib on the outgrowth of metastatic breast cancer cells to the brain. *J Natl Cancer Inst* 2008; 100:1092–1103.
84. Lin NU, Diéras V, Paul D *et al*. Multicenter phase II study of lapatinib in patients with brain metastases from HER-2-positive breast cancer. *Clin Cancer Res* 2009; 15:1452–1459.
85. Goss P, Smith I, O'Shaugnessy J *et al*. Results of a randomized, double-blind, multicenter, placebo-controlled study of adjuvant lapatinib in women with early-stage erbB2-overexpressing breast cancer. Abstract # S4–7. Presented at San Antonio Breast Cancer Conference, San Antonio (USA), 2011.
86. Burstein HJ, Sun Y, Dirix LY. Neratinib, an irreversible ErbB receptor tyrosine kinase inhibitor, in patients with advanced ErbB2-positive breast cancer. *J Clin Oncol* 2010; 28:1301–1307.
87. Martin M, Bonneterre J, Geyer CE Jr *et al*. A Phase 2, randomized, open-label study of neratinib (HKI-272) vs. lapatinib plus capecitabine for 2nd/3rd-line treatment of HER-2+ locally advanced or metastatic breast cancer. Abstract # S5–7. Presented at San Antonio Breast Cancer Conference, San Antonio (USA), 2011.
88. Saura C, Martin M, Moroose R *et al*. Safety of neratinib (HKI-272) in combination with capecitabine in patients with solid tumors: A phase 1/2 Study. *Ann Oncol* 2010; 21(suppl 4):Abstract 147P.65.
89. Baselga J, Swain SM. Novel anticancer targets: revisiting ERBB2 and discovering ERBB3. *Nat Rev Cancer* 2009; 9:463–475.
90. Franklin MC, Carey KD, Vajdos FF, Leahy DJ, de Vos AM, Sliwkowski MX. Insights into ErbB signaling from the structure of the ErbB2-pertuzumab complex. *Cancer Cell* 2004; 5:317–328.
91. Nahta R, Hung M-C, Esteva FJ. The HER-2-targeting antibodies trastuzumab and pertuzumab synergistically inhibit the survival of breast cancer cells. *Cancer Res* 2004; 64:2343–2346.

92. Scheuer W, Friess T, Burtscher H, Bossenmaier B, Endl J, Hasmann M. Strongly enhanced antitumor activity of trastuzumab and pertuzumab combination treatment on HER-2-positive human xenograft tumor models. *Cancer Res* 2009; 69:9330–9336.
93. Arpino G, Gutierrez C, Weiss H *et al.* Treatment of human epidermal growth factor receptor 2-overexpressing breast cancer xenografts with multiagent HER-targeted therapy. *J Natl Cancer Inst* 2007; 99:694–705.
94. Gianni L, Lladó A, Bianchi G *et al.* Open-label, phase II, multicenter, randomized study of the efficacy and safety of two dose levels of Pertuzumab, a human epidermal growth factor receptor 2 dimerization inhibitor, in patients with human epidermal growth factor receptor 2-negative metastatic breast cancer. *J Clin Oncol* 2010; 28:1131–1137.
95. Baselga J, Gelmon KA, Verma S *et al.* Phase II trial of pertuzumab and trastuzumab in patients with human epidermal growth factor receptor 2-positive metastatic breast cancer that progressed during prior trastuzumab therapy. *J Clin Oncol* 2010; 28:1138–1144.
96. Baselga J, Cortés J, Kim SB *et al.* CLEOPATRA Study Group. Pertuzumab plus trastuzumab plus docetaxel for metastatic breast cancer. *N Engl J Med* 2012; 366:109–119.
97. Gianni L, Pienkowski T, Im Y-H *et al.* Neoadjuvant pertuzumab (P) and trastuzumab (H): antitumor and safety analysis of a randomized phase II study ('NeoSphere'). *Cancer Res* 2010; 70(suppl 24):Abstract S3–2.
98. Schneeweiss A, Chia S, Hickish T *et al.* Neoadjuvant pertuzumab and trastuzumab concurrent or sequential with an anthracycline-containing or concurrent with an anthracycline-free standard regimen: a randomized phase II study (TRYPHAENA). *Cancer Res* 2011; 71(suppl 24):Abstract S5–6.
99. Lenihan D, Suter T, Brammer M, Neate C, Ross G, Baselga J. Pooled analysis of cardiac safety in patients with cancer treated with pertuzumab. *Ann Oncol* 2012; 23:791–800 [Epub 2011 Jun 10].
100. Lee KF, Simon H, Chen H, Bates B, Hung MC, Hauser C. Requirement for neuregulin receptor erbB2 in neural and cardiac development. *Nature* 1995; 378:394–398.
101. Press MF, Cordon-Cardo C, Slamon DJ. Expression of the HER-2/neu proto-oncogene in normal human adult and fetal tissues. *Oncogene* 1990; 5:953–962.
102. Bates SE, Amiri-Kordestani L, Giaccone G. Drug development: portals of discovery. *Clin Cancer Res* 2012; 18:23–32.
103. Chari RV, Martell BA, Gross JL *et al.* Immunoconjugates containing novel maytansinoids: promising anticancer drugs. *Cancer Res* 1992; 52:127–131.
104. Remillard S, Rebhun LI, Howie GS *et al.* Antimitotic activity of the potent tumor inhibitor maytansine. *Science* 1975; 189:1002–1005.
105. Erickson HK, Park PU, Widdison WC *et al.* Antibody-maytansinoid conjugates are activated in targeted cancer cells by lysosomal degradation and linker-dependent intracellular processing. *Cancer Res* 2006; 66:4426–4433.
106. Junttila T, Fields C, Li G *et al.* Trastuzumab-mertansine (T-DM1) retains all the mechanisms of action (MOA) of trastuzumab and is extremely effective in combination with docetaxel. Presented at 20th EORTC-NCI-AACR Symposium on Molecular Targets and Cancer Therapeutics, 2008. Geneva, Switzerland.
107. Lewis Phillips GD, Li G, Dugger DL *et al.* Targeting HER-2 -positive breast cancer with trastuzumab-DM1, an antibody-cytotoxic drug conjugate. *Cancer Res* 2008; 68:9280–9290.
108. Krop IE, Beeram M, Modi S *et al.* Phase I study of trastuzumab-DM1, an HER-2 antibody-drug conjugate, given every 3 weeks to patients with HER-2-positive metastatic breast cancer. *J Clin Oncol* 2010; 28:2698–2704.
109. Burris HA III, Rugo HS, Vukelja SJ *et al.* Phase II study of the antibody drug conjugate trastuzumab-DM1 for the treatment of human epidermal growth factor receptor 2 (HER-2)-positive breast cancer after prior HER-2 directed therapy. *J Clin Oncol* 2011; 29:398–405.
110. Perez EA, Dirix L, Kocsis J *et al.* Efficacy and safety of trastuzumab-DM1 vs trastuzumab plus docetaxel in HER2-positive metastatic breast cancer patients with no prior chemotherapy for metastatic disease: preliminary results of a randomized, multicenter, open-label phase 2 study (TDM4450G). *Ann Oncol* 2010; 21:Abstract LBA3.
111. Verma S, Miles D, Gianni L *et al*; EMILIA Study Group. Trastuzumab emtansine for HER2-positive advanced breast cancer. *N Engl J Med* 2012; 367:1783–1791.
112. Baselga J. Targeting the phosphoinositide-3 (PI3) kinase pathway in breast cancer. *Oncologist* 2011; 16:12–19 (review).

113. Serra V, Scaltriti M, Prudkin L *et al.* PI3K inhibition results in enhanced HER signaling and acquired ERK dependency in HER2-overexpressing breast cancer. *Oncogene* 2011; 30:2547–2557.
114. Dave B, Migliaccio I, Gutierrez MC *et al.* Loss of phosphatase and tensin homolog or phosphoinositol-3 kinase activation and response to trastuzumab or lapatinib in human epidermal growth factor receptor 2-overexpressing locally advanced breast cancers. *J Clin Oncol* 2011; 29:166–173.
115. O'Brien NA, Browne BC, Chow L *et al.* Activated phosphoinositide 3-kinase/AKT signaling confers resistance to trastuzumab but not lapatinib. *Mol Cancer Ther* 2010; 9:1489–1502.
116. Nagata Y, Lan KH, Zhou X *et al.* PTEN activation contributes to tumor inhibition by trastuzumab, and loss of PTEN predicts trastuzumab resistance in patients. *Cancer Cell* 2004; 6:117–127.
117. Esteva FJ, Guo H, Zhang S *et al.* PTEN, PIK3CA, p-AKT, and p-p70S6K status: association with trastuzumab response and survival in patients with HER-2-positive metastatic breast cancer. *Am J Pathol* 2010; 177:1647–1656.
118. Razis E, Bobos M, Kotoula V *et al.* Evaluation of the association of PIK3CA mutations and PTEN loss with efficacy of trastuzumab therapy in metastatic breast cancer. *Breast Cancer Res Treat* 2011; 128: 447–456.
119. Wang L, Zhang Q, Zhang J *et al.* PI3K pathway activation results in low efficacy of both trastuzumab and lapatinib. *BMC Cancer* 2011; 11:248. doi: 10.1186/1471-2407-11-248.
120. Morrow PK, Wulf GM, Ensor J *et al.* Phase I/II study of trastuzumab in combination with everolimus (RAD001) in patients with HER-2-overexpressing metastatic breast cancer who progressed on trastuzumab-based therapy. *J Clin Oncol* 2011; 29:3126–3132.
121. Neckers L, Ivy SP. Heat shock protein 90. *Curr Opin Oncol* 2003; 15:419–424 (review).
122. Citri A, Kochupurakkal BS, Yarden Y. The achilles heel of ErbB-2/HER2: regulation by the Hsp90 chaperone machine and potential for pharmacological intervention. *Cell Cycle* 2004; 1:51–60 (review).
123. Raja SM, Clubb RJ, Bhattacharyya M *et al.* A combination of trastuzumab and 17-AAG induces enhanced ubiquitinylation and lysosomal pathway-dependent ErbB2 degradation and cytotoxicity in ErbB2-overexpressing breast cancer cells. *Cancer Biol Ther* 2008; 7:1630–1640.
124. Whitesell L, Mimnaugh EG, De Cost B *et al.* Inhibition of heat shock protein Hsp90-pp60v-src heteroprotein complex formation by benzoquinone ansamycins: essential role for stress proteins in oncogenic transformation. *Proc Natl Acad Sci USA* 1994; 91:8324–8328.
125. Basso A, Solit DB, Munster PN *et al.* Ansamycin antibiotics inhibit Akt activation and cyclin D expression in breast cancer cells that overexpress HER-2. *Oncogene* 2002; 21:1159–1166.
126. Workman P, Burrows F, Neckers L, Rosen N. Drugging the cancer chaperone HSP90: combinatorial therapeutic exploitation of oncogene addiction and tumor stress. *Ann N Y Acad Sci* 2007; 1113: 202–216.
127. Chandarlapaty S, Scaltriti M, Angelini P *et al.* Inhibitors of HSP90 block p95-HER2 signaling in Trastuzumab-resistant tumors and suppress their growth. *Oncogene* 2010; 29:325–334.
128. Arteaga CL. Why is this effective HSP90 inhibitor not being developed in HER2+ breast cancer? *Clin Cancer Res* 2011; 17:4919–4921.
129. Banerji U, O'Donnell A, Scurr M *et al.* Phase I pharmacokinetic and pharmacodynamic study of 17-allylamino, 17-demethoxygeldanamycin in patients with advanced malignancies. *J Clin Oncol* 2005; 23:4152–4161.
130. Goetz MP, Toft D, Reid J *et al.* Phase I trial of 17-allylamino-17-demethoxygeldanamycin in patients with advanced cancer. *J Clin Oncol* 2005; 23:1078–1087.
131. Solit DB, Ivy P, Kopil C *et al.* Phase I trial of 17-allylamino-17-demethoxygeldanamycin in patients with advanced cancer. *Clin Cancer Res* 2007; 13:1775–1782.
132. Modi S, Stopeck AT, Gordon MS *et al.* Combination of trastuzumab and tanespimycin (17-AAG, KOS-953) is safe and active in trastuzumab-refractory HER-2 overexpressing breast cancer: a phase I dose-escalation study. *J Clin Oncol* 2007; 25:5410–5417.
133. Modi S, Stopeck A, Linden H *et al.* HSP90 inhibition is effective in breast cancer: a phase II trial of tanespimycin (17-AAG) plus trastuzumab in patients with HER-2-positive metastatic breast cancer progressing on trastuzumab. *Clin Cancer Res* 2011; 17:5132–5139.
134. Scaltriti M, Serra V, Normant E *et al.* Antitumor activity of the Hsp90 inhibitor IPI-504 in HER-2 -positive trastuzumab-resistant breast cancer. *Mol Cancer Ther* 2011; 10:817–824.
135. Ladjemi MZ, Jacot W, Chardès T, Pèlegrin A, Navarro-Teulon I. Anti-HER2 vaccines: new prospects for breast cancer therapy. *Cancer Immunol Immunother* 2010; 59:1295–1312 (review).

136. Disis ML, Schiffman K. Cancer vaccines targeting the HER2/neu oncogenic protein. *Semin Oncol* 2001; 6:12–20 (review).
137. Disis ML, Bernhard H, Shiota FM *et al.* Granulocyte-macrophage colony-stimulating factor: an effective adjuvant for protein and peptide-based vaccines. *Blood* 1996; 88:202–210.
138. Disis ML, Cheever MA. HER-2/neu oncogenic protein: issues in vaccine development. *Crit Rev Immunol* 1998; 18:37–45 (review).
139. Peoples GE, Gurney JM, Hueman MT *et al.* Clinical trial results of a HER-2/neu (E75) vaccine to prevent recurrence in high-risk breast cancer patients. *J Clin Oncol* 2005; 23:7536–7545.
140. Mittendorf EA, Storrer CE, Shriver CD, Ponniah S, Peoples GE. Investigating the combination of trastuzumab and HER-2/neu peptide vaccines for the treatment of breast cancer. *Ann Surg Oncol* 2006; 13:1085–1098.
141. Disis ML, Wallace DR, Gooley TA *et al.* Concurrent trastuzumab and HER-2/neu-specific vaccination in patients with metastatic breast cancer. *J Clin Oncol* 2009; 27:4685–4692.
142. Emens LA, Asquith JM, Leatherman JM *et al.* Timed sequential treatment with cyclophosphamide, doxorubicin, and an allogeneic granulocyte-macrophage colony-stimulating factor-secreting breast tumor vaccine: a chemotherapy dose-ranging factorial study of safety and immune activation. *J Clin Oncol* 2009; 27:5911–5918.
143. Jacob JB, Kong YC, Nalbantoglu I, Snower DP, Wei WZ. Tumor regression following DNA vaccination and regulatory T cell depletion in neu transgenic mice leads to an increased risk for autoimmunity. *J Immunol* 2009; 182:5873–5881.
144. Isakoff SJ, Baselga J. Trastuzumab-DM1: building a chemotherapy-free road in the treatment of human epidermal growth factor receptor 2-positive breast cancer. *J Clin Oncol* 2011; 29:351–354.
145. Eichhorn PJ, Gili M, Scaltriti M *et al.* Phosphatidylinositol 3-kinase hyperactivation results in lapatinib resistance that is reversed by the mTOR/phosphatidylinositol 3-kinase inhibitor NVP-BEZ235. *Cancer Res* 2008; 68:9221–9230.
146. Untch M, Fasching PA, Konecny GE *et al.* Pathologic complete response after neoadjuvant chemotherapy plus trastuzumab predicts favorable survival in human epidermal growth factor receptor 2-overexpressing breast cancer: results from the TECHNO trial of the AGO and GBG study groups. *J Clin Oncol* 2011; 29:3351–3357.
147. Bardia A, Greenup R, Moy B, Smith B, Baselga J. Pathological complete remission after neoadjuvant chemotherapy predicts improved survival in the various breast cancer subtypes: systematic review and meta-analyses. Presented at AACR Advances in Breast Cancer Research, San Francisco, CA, 2011.
148. Ellis MJ, Tao Y, Luo J *et al.* Outcome prediction for estrogen receptor-positive breast cancer based on postneoadjuvant endocrine therapy tumor characteristics. *J Natl Cancer Inst* 2008; 100:1380–1388.
149. Gamez C, Flamen P, Holmes E *et al.* FDG-PET/CT for early prediction of response to neoadjuvant lapatinib, trastuzumab, and their combination in HER-2-positive breast cancer patients: the Neo-ALTTO study results. Abstract #5013. Presented at European Multidisciplinary Cancer Congress, Stockholm, 2011.
150. Flores LM, Kindelberger DW, Ligon AH *et al.* Improving the yield of circulating tumour cells facilitates molecular characterisation and recognition of discordant HER-2 amplification in breast cancer. *Br J Cancer* 2010; 102:1495–1502.
151. Wülfing P, Borchard J, Buerger H *et al.* HER-2-positive circulating tumor cells indicate poor clinical outcome in stage I to III breast cancer patients. *Clin Cancer Res* 2006; 12:1715–1720.
152. DiMasi JA, Grabowski HG. Economics of new oncology drug development. *J Clin Oncol* 2007; 25: 209–216.

5

Chemotherapy as targeted therapy

R. Audet, R. Duchnowska, C. Shen, S. Willis, G.W. Sledge Jr., B. Leyland-Jones

INTRODUCTION

In the metastatic context, selection of specific breast cancer treatment currently depends on hormone-receptor and HER2 status. For those patients who are non-responsive to endocrine therapy or have tumors negative for hormone receptors, standard chemotherapy remains the most common treatment option with single agent regimens usually consisting of either anthracyclines, taxanes, cyclophosphamide, fluorouracile, capecitabine, vinorelbine, or gemcitabine [1, 2]. Unfortunately, there is no specific recommendation at present for second-line treatment or further chemotherapy as no particular regimen has been shown to offer greater efficacy [3]. In fact, from the 60% of patients with early-stage breast cancer that will receive adjuvant chemotherapy, only 2–15% will ultimately derive benefit from treatment, while all treated patients will be exposed to toxic side-effects [4].

The primary objective of pharmacogenomics is to develop markers able to address specific aspects of response and/or toxicity and help in the individualization of breast cancer therapy. Biomarkers can be broadly categorized either as prognostic when solely associated with clinical outcome, and predictive when associated with the effectiveness of a specific drug. A prognostic marker is a unique molecular feature or set of features assembled as a signature, which can separate populations of patients based on disease outcome in the absence of treatment or despite a non-specific treatment. A predictive marker is, on the other hand, a unique molecular feature or signature of features that can separate patient populations based on clinical outcome derived from a specific targeted therapy. When a predictive marker has been properly validated, it can help to identify patients most likely to expect to benefit, or be less susceptible to suffer side effects, from a particular therapy.

The quest for reliable predictive biomarkers for cytotoxic agents has been, and will certainly remain, a long and challenging enterprise. As we gain a better understanding of the weaknesses of the available methodologies, it is becoming increasingly evident that each step in the analysis process is critical with regard to accuracy, reproducibility, and predictive

Robert Audet, PhD, V M Institute of Research, Montréal, Quebec, Canada.

Renata Duchnowska, MD, PhD, Military Institute of Medicine, Warsaw, Poland.

Changyu Shen, PhD, Division of Biostatistics, Indiana University School of Medicine, Indianapolis, Indiana, USA.

Scooter Willis, PhD, Edith Sanford Breast Cancer Research, Sioux Falls, South Dakota, USA.

George W. Sledge, Jr., MD, Professor, Department of Medicine; Chief, Division of Oncology, Stanford University School of Medicine, Palo Alto, California, USA.

Brian Leyland-Jones, MD, PhD, Edith Sanford Breast Cancer Research, Sioux Falls, South Dakota, USA.

value of new markers or signatures [5]. In order to minimize inaccuracies, complementary techniques have been selected in parallel to assess the usefulness of these biomarkers in predicting the response of an individual patient to a specific therapy.

Three different strategies were used to identify markers or signatures for each cytotoxic agent used in the Center of Excellence (COE) breast cancer retrospective cohorts.

1. Based on the concept that potential biomarkers have a better chance of being linked to a clinical response, a set of biomarkers were identified as either targets of a particular cytotoxic agent or determinants of its metabolism (Table 5.1). Gene copy number, or protein expression, of some of these selected markers, was evaluated using fluorescent *in situ* hybridization (FISH) and immunohistochemistry (IHC), respectively.
2. Using an mRNA expression profiling microarray-based assay (WG-DASL; Whole Genome cDNA-mediated Annealing, Selection extension and Ligation), genes that show a high differential expression between groups of patients with either a good or bad prognosis for a particular chemotherapeutic agent were characterized with univariate methods.
3. A dataset containing gene identifiers and corresponding WG-DASL gene expression values was uploaded to the Ingenuity application (*http://www.broadinstitute.org/gsea/index.jsp*) and mapped to its corresponding object in Ingenuity's Knowledge Base. Sets of genes grouped either by similar functional attributes, common transcription factor-driven expression, or chromosomal proximity, that were most significant to the clinical outcome data, were identified using Ingenuity's Knowledge Base.

PATIENT SELECTION

Patients included in this study were all adult females over 18 years of age with pathologically confirmed breast cancer and locally advanced or metastatic disease treated with one or more of the following treatment regimens.

Cohort A: Doxorubicin 60 mg/m^2 and cyclophosphamide 600 mg/m^2 day 1 of every 21-day cycle
Cohort B: Capecitabine 1000 mg/m^2 BID days 1–14 of a 21-day cycle
Cohort C: Vinorelbine 25 mg/m^2 days 1, 8, 15 of every 28-day cycle
Cohort D: Gemcitabine 1000 mg/m^2 days 1, 8, 15 of every 28-day cycle

Archival formalin-fixed paraffin embedded (FFPE) blocks were obtained, sectioned, and the resulting slices were either mounted on glass slides for FISH and IHC analysis or kept in RNase-free tubes for RNA extraction and further WG-DASL or polymerase chain reaction (PCR)-based analysis.

The main clinical endpoints were time to progression (TTP) and progression-free survival (PFS). TTP was defined as the time from treatment to disease progression. PFS was defined as the time from treatment to disease progression or death, whichever occurred earlier.

ANALYSES FOR THE CENTER OF EXCELLENCE (COE) STUDIES

Overview of analyses per protocol and treatment cohort

Selected markers and the corresponding methodologies to evaluate them are summarized in Table 5.1 for each of the treatments of the COE cohorts. The biomarker selection rationale, along with a summary of results for each cytotoxic treatment, is given in the following sections.

Table 5.1 Overview of the selected analyses for each treatment cohort

Protocol	*FISH*[1]			*Immunohistochemistry*[2]			*WG-DASL*[3]	*Potential markers for qRT-PCR*
COE-01 and COE-05								
Cohort A: AC	TOP2			HER2			√	ALDH1A1, HER1, HER2, HER3, TOP2A,
Cohort B: Capecitabine	DHFR	TYMP	TYMS				√	DHFR, DPYD, TYMP, TYMS
Cohort C: Vinorelbine							√	STMN1, TUBB3,
Cohort D: Gemcitabine				ENT	DCK	CNT	√	CNT, DCK, ENT, RRM1

Abbreviations: AC: Adriamycin® (doxorubicin) and cyclophosphamide, ALDH1A1: aldehyde dehydrogenase 1, CNT: concentrative nucleoside transporter, COE: Center of Excellence, DCK: deoxycytidine kinase, DHFR: dihydrofolate reductase, DPYD: dihydropyrimidine dehydrogenase, ENT: equilibrative nucleoside transporter, FISH: fluorescent *in situ* hybridization, HER: human epidermal growth factor receptor, qRT-PCR: quantitative real time polymerase chain reaction, RRM: ribonucleotide reductase M, STMN1: stathmin 1, TOP2A: DNA topoisomerase-2-alpha, TUBB3: tubulin beta 3, TYMP: thymidine phosphorylase, TYMS: thymidylate synthase, WG-DASL: Whole Genome cDNA-mediated-Annealing, Selection, extension and Ligation.

[1] FISH probes developed by Dako (Glostrup, Denmark) were used on 5-µm FFPE tissue slices to investigate TOP2A, DHFR, TYMP or TYMS gene copy number. Hybridization signals were evaluated in at least 60 morphologically intact and non-overlapping nuclei. The TOP2A genes to reference sequence ratio was considered deleted <0.8, normal ≥ 0.8 and <2.0, and amplified ≥ 2.0. The DHFR, TYMP and TYMS gene copy number was dichotomized by the median.

[2] Antibodies for hENT, hCNT and dCK were synthesized in Dr. John Mackey's lab and used according to established protocols [6, 7].

[3] Total RNA was extracted from 5-µm thick FFPE sections using the EPICENTRE QuickExtract™ kit and converted into cDNA before being hybridized to Whole-Genome-cDNA-mediated Annealing, Selection extension and Ligation BeadChips (Illumina, Inc., San Diego, CA, USA) according to the manufacturer's instructions. The signals were processed with the Bead-Studio Gene Expression Module (Illumina, Inc., San Diego, CA, USA).

Statistical analysis

Normalization

There are many sources of noise in microarray data. The dye, scanner, arrays, and pin groups used to print the spot can all affect the expression level observed. This made normalization a critical step in order to eliminate bias. However, over-normalization may eliminate true biological signals as well. In consideration of both aspects, median normalization was used throughout our analyses where the median of signals from different arrays is normalized to be the same.

Comparison step

For binary outcome (response vs. non-response), significance analysis of microarray (SAM) and prediction analysis of microarray (PAM) were used for feature selection and the control of false discovery rate (FDR). These two approaches allow FDR to be controlled by estimating the null distribution of the test statistic (e.g. T-statistic) through permutation or parametric modeling. The estimate is relatively robust to deviation from standard normal, which is partially due to the correlation among those signals. The Cox proportional regression model was used for the survival-type of outcome (e.g. TTP and PFS) and to control the FDR.

Gene ontology analysis

To evaluate gene functions and categories defined by various criteria, gene ontology (GO) offers a convenient platform (*http://www.geneontology.org/*). For each of the three types of GO terms (molecular function, biological process and cellular component), hypergeometric distribution can be used to test the over/under-representation of each term for the genes displaying differential expression between groups. A significant *P*-value then suggests that the very feature that defines the groups (e.g. response or non-response) might be correlated with the term under consideration (e.g. a specific biological function).

An alternative approach is gene set enrichment analysis (GSEA software: *http://www.broadinstitute.org/gsea/index.jsp*). In GSEA, a set of prespecified genes was constructed based on certain biological rationales (e.g. involved in the same biological process or pathways). The analysis seeks to assess whether or not the gene expression level for the set as a whole (e.g. summary measure of expression level of genes in the set) differs between the comparison groups. It has the advantage of detecting a set of small signals that would otherwise be difficult to detect.

Marker selection rationale for cohort A: doxorubicin and cyclophosphamide

Molecular pharmacology and mechanisms of action

Cyclophosphamide is a prodrug that undergoes activation through phase I metabolism via the enzymes CYP2B6, CYP3A4, CYP3A5 and CYP2C9 into 4-hydroxy-cyclophosphamide, the active metabolite responsible for cyclophosphamide's alkylating properties [8, 9]. This molecule can be inactivated through a phase II conjugation with a thiol or sulfate via glutathione S-transferases (GSTs) or oxidized by the enzyme aldehyde dehydrogenase 1 (ALDH1) into carboxyphosphamide [10].

A correlation between single nucleotide polymorphism in the activating enzyme *CYP3A4* or the metabolizing enzyme *GST1* and clinical outcome was suggested by small studies in breast cancer [11–13] but it is only recently that an association between small nucleotide polymorphism and cyclophosphamide efficacy has been observed in a larger cohort [14]. Although conceptually interesting, a direct link between the expression of these enzymes and clinical efficacy of cyclophosphamide-based chemotherapeutic regimens remains to be established.

The cancer stem cell hypothesis has fueled much research on *ALDH1* as a marker of breast cancer stem cells [15] but it was also shown to be a predictor of response to cyclophosphamide in breast cancer patients [16]. Although the number of patients was small, the authors were able to show that the therapeutic outcome of cyclophosphamide-based chemotherapy corresponded to cellular ALDH1A1 levels in 77% of cases [16]. Indirect evidence is also available from many *in vitro* studies showing that ALDH1A1 is directly linked to sensitivity to cyclophosphamide, consistent with its role in cyclophosphamide metabolism [15, 17–20].

The anthracycline doxorubicin has been one of the most widely used agents in the treatment of breast cancer for the past quarter century. Anthracyclines have three principal mechanisms of actions:

1. They intercalate themselves between base pairs of DNA/RNA strands thereby inhibiting DNA and RNA synthesis.
2. They enhance the catalytic oxidation–reduction reactions.
3. They inhibit topoisomerase II alpha (*TOP2A*).

Although evidence suggests that anthracycline-based regimens are significantly more efficacious than non anthracycline-based regimens in *HER2* positive patients but not *HER2* negative patients, some studies have demonstrated that response to treatment in this group is not uniform [21]. This has led to the postulation that anthracyclines target *TOP2A*. With its gene neighboring the *HER2* gene on chromosome 17q12–21, *TOP2A* may be the modulator of response to therapy. This interest was sparked by the finding that the *TOP2A* gene is frequently co-amplified with *HER2* [22–24]. However, this notion is complicated by the fact that *TOP2A* amplification does not strongly correlate with TOP2A protein expression [25–27]. Besides *TOP2A* amplification, some authors have observed *TOP2A* deletions and found incidence levels ranging from 16% to 43% in *HER2* amplified tumors [22, 28, 29].

Although recent data show that *TOP2A* is also amplified in 27% of *HER2* negative tumors [30], previous data showing that *TOP2A* aberrations are found almost exclusively in *HER2* amplified tumors, and that both *TOP2A* deletions and amplifications can be found in the same tumor, led to the theory of a cascade-type effect at 17q12–21 [31]. These authors propose that *HER2* amplification is the first step in a series leading to an increased rate of *TOP2A* aberrations and possibly other surrounding genes. Coherent with the observed higher level of amplification for *HER2* compared to *TOP2A*, Nielsen *et al.* recently showed that co-amplification of *HER2* and *TOP2A* is not the main mechanism behind aberrations seen in these genes and that different mechanisms may be involved [32].

Attempts to come up with a gene signature predicting benefits from anthracycline-based therapy are currently being pursued and recent publications suggest that such a panel of biomarkers will necessarily involve many aberrant genes leading to altered protein expression and cellular regulation [33]. Recently, strategies to overcome the inherent noise in microarray data were developed with the selection of genes with common features or their relation in the intracellular network [34].

The present research aim is twofold:

1. To shed some light on possible links between clinical efficacy of AC and *HER2* and *TOP2A* gene aberrations as well as their gene expression levels.
2. To determine if a specific gene expression signature could be used as predictive marker for treatment outcome.

Results summary for cohort A: doxorubicin and cyclophosphamide

Sixty adult female patients with pathologically confirmed locally advanced or metastatic breast cancer were treated with doxorubicin 60 mg/m^2 and cyclophosphamide 600 mg/m^2 day 1 of every 21-day cycle. Archival FFPE specimens, taken before chemotherapy, were

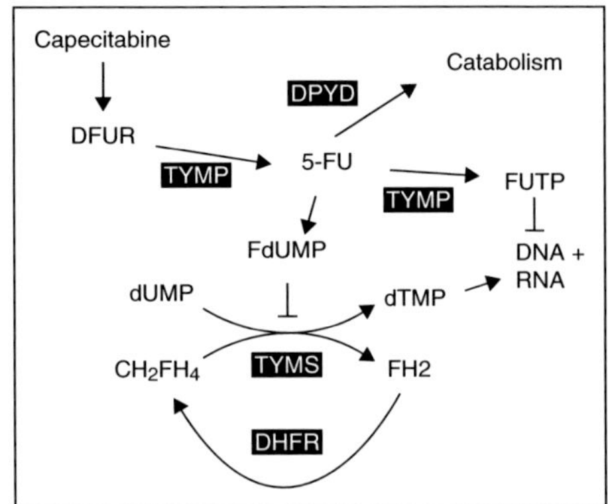

Figure 5.1 Pathway of capecitabine metabolism and catabolism. Abbreviations: CH_2FH_4, 5–10 methylenetetrahydrofolate; DFUR, 5′-deoxy-5-fluorouridine; DHFR, dihydrofolate reductase; DPYD, dihydropyrimidine dehydrogenase; dTMP, deoxythymidine-5′-monophosphate; dUMP, deoxyuridine-5′-monophosphate; FdUMP, 5-flurodeoxyuridine-5′-monophosphate; FH2, dihydrofolate; 5-FU, fluorouracil; FUTP, fluorouridine triphosphate; TYMP, thymidine phosphorylase; TYMS, thymidylate synthase.

used to evaluate *TOP2A* gene status by FISH, *HER2* gene expression by IHC, and WG-DASL gene expression as described in the previous section.

Full statistical analysis is currently underway and will be subsequently published, but interim results suggest that *TOP2A* FISH gene copy number could be useful to identify patient populations most likely to benefit from an anthracycline-based therapy. These results should also shed some light on the link between *TOP2A* gene aberrations and altered gene expression.

Interim univariate expression analysis of key genes is also underway and will be published shortly but does not seem as promising as GSEA in helping to predict clinical outcome. GSEA clustering by functional attributes, chromosomal location or common transcription factor-driven gene expression provides important insights into complex gene expression changes related to the efficacy of chemotherapeutic agents. This novel approach holds the promise of facilitating the identification of gene sets enriched in tumors of patients with either more favorable or poorer outcomes when treated with anthracycline regimens.

Marker selection rationale for cohort B: capecitabine

Molecular pharmacology and mechanisms of action

The fluoropyrimidine nucleoside analogue fluorouracil (5-FU) was originally developed as a cytotoxic agent over 50 years ago and is the standard treatment for a wide range of common solid tumors, including breast cancer. Attempts to increase the efficacy and tolerability of fluoropyrimidine treatment have led to the development of capecitabine (Xeloda™), a prodrug transformed into 5-FU preferentially in tumors (Figure 5.1). Capecitabine is now often used either alone or in combination with other drugs but, unfortunately, reliable methods for the selection of patients with the best chance of benefiting from capecitabine-based treatments are still lacking.

Capecitabine is activated at the tumor site by the enzyme thymidine phosphorylase (TYMP) [35], which takes advantage of the fact that this enzyme is more highly expressed in tumor tissue [36], including breast cancer [37]. Capecitabine and its intermediate metabolite, 5′-deoxy-5-fluorouridine (5′-DFUR) are not cytotoxic but become effective only after conversion to 5-FU by TYMP as well as further transformations into fluorodeoxyuridine monophosphate (FdUMP) and fluorouridine triphosphate (FUTP)

[35]. Inhibition of the enzyme thymidylate synthase (TYMS) by FdUMP is considered to be the main mechanism of action of fluoropyrimidine, including capecitabine [38].

TYMS is an important enzyme in pyrimidine metabolism which is crucial for *de novo* thymidine nucleotide synthesis used for DNA replication and cellular division [39]. Inhibition of TYMS occurs as a result of the formation of an inactive ternary covalent complex between TYMS, FdUMP, and 5–10 methylenetetrahydrofolate (CH_2FH_4). The stability of this ternary complex is highly dependent on the availability of CH_2FH_4 or one of its polylglutamates [40, 41]. Dihydrofolate reductase (DHFR) is a key enzyme involved in folate metabolism and plays a role in the *de novo* pathway of pyrimidine biosynthesis that has been linked to the modulation of fluoropyrimidine treatments [42, 43].

Dihydropyrimidine dehydrogenase (DPYD) is the enzyme responsible for the first and rate-limiting step in the catabolic conversion of 5-FU to inactive metabolites and decreases 5-FU levels within cells [44–46]. Several studies have underlined the role of *DPYD* deficiency in the development of severe 5-FU toxicity and conversely *DPYD* over-expression is associated with resistance to these therapies [47]. Both elevated *DPYD* gene copy number and mRNA expression have been linked to increased resistance to capecitabine and other 5-FU-based treatments in several human cells lines including breast [48].

Since DPYD is rate-limiting for the catabolic pathway and TYMP is key to the production of active capecitabine metabolites, the TYMP/DPYD ratio has been frequently used to correlate with capecitabine or 5-FU efficacy. It was first shown that a high TYMP to DPYD ratio correlated with high capecitabine efficacy and conversely a low TYMP/DPYD ratio was linked to resistance in a large number of xenograft models including breast [49]. Recent IHC data have shown that a higher TYMP/DPYD ratio correlates with a better clinical response in a small cohort of breast cancer patients treated with capecitabine monotherapy [50].

Similarly, RT-PCR analysis of tumors from 22 breast cancer patients revealed that the patients expressing high levels of *TYMS* and *DPYD* were resistant to 5-FU, as opposed to the patients expressing low levels of *TYMS* and *DPYD*, who were sensitive to this compound [51]. Using IHC, it was shown that high levels of *TYMP* expression in tumors was a significant prognostic indicator of 5′-DFUR efficacy in breast cancer patients [52].

Therefore, the fluoropyrimidine pathway enzymes, TYMP, TYMS, DPYD and DHFR, were selected as potential candidate biomarkers that could be used to predict tumor response to capecitabine. Efforts have been made to select assays that would be easily accessible to clinicians in order to correlate gene copy number and gene expression profiles with disease state, therapy, and drug response.

Results summary for cohort B: capecitabine

Newly developed FISH probes (Dako, Glostrup, Denmark) were used on 5-μm FFPE tissue slices to investigate TYMS, DHFR and TYMP gene copy number. Hybridization signals were evaluated using either the ratio of red signals for TYMS, DHFR or TYMP to green signals for a reference sequence on the same chromosome or only the green signal from genes in at least 60 morphologically intact and non-overlapping nuclei. As these new probes have not been fully characterized, a threshold (as for the TOP2A FISH probes) was not applied, but the results were categorized into high versus low gene copy number by the median.

TYMS is the primary target of capecitabine. Interim results presented at the San Antonio Breast Cancer Symposium in 2011 show that higher *TYMS* gene copy number was significantly associated with a higher hazard ratio (HR) of both PFS and TTP in the overall patient population as well as in the *ER+* and *HER2–* subpopulations (Table 5.2 and Figure 5.2). *TYMS* gene copy number was also shown to be significantly correlated with its gene expression by DASL suggesting that multiple gene copies induce an increase in gene expression (Table 5.3). Although higher *TYMS* gene expression measured with DASL was also associated with increased HR both in the overall population, and in the *ER+* and *HER2–* subpopulations, they failed to reach the statistical significance level (Table 5.4 and Figure 5.3). These

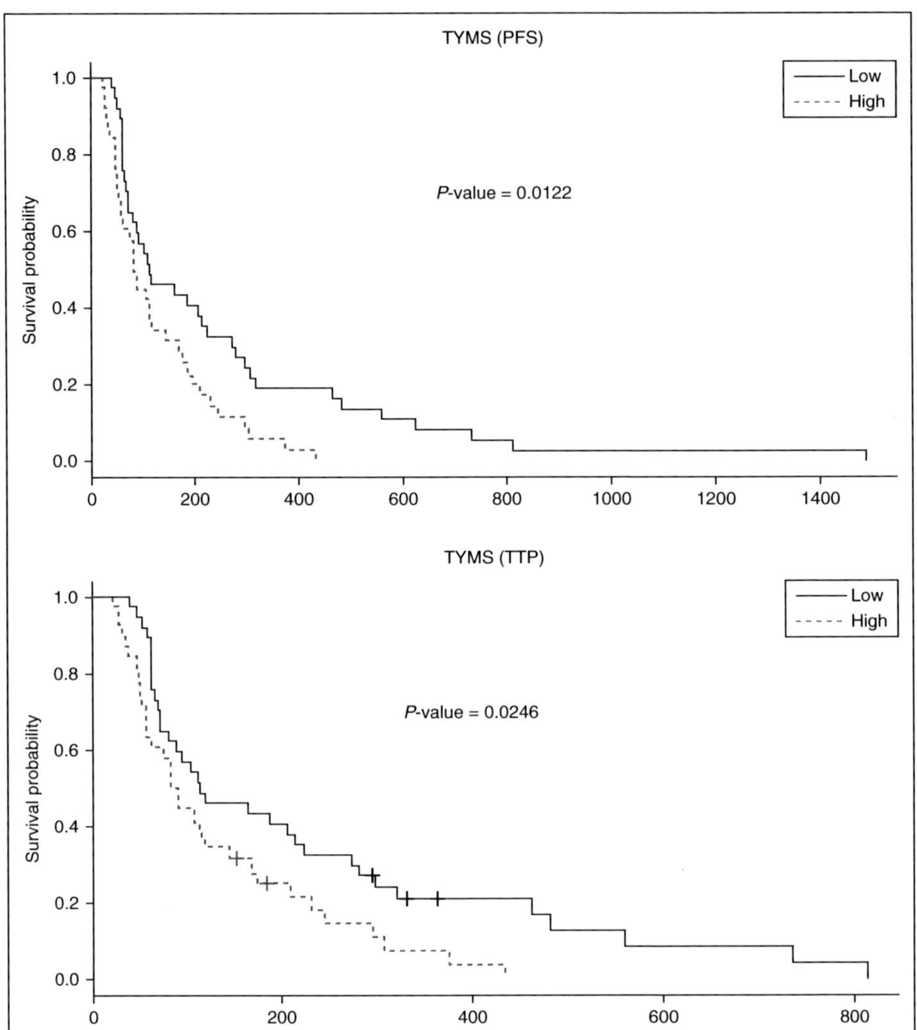

Figure 5.2 Progression-free survival (PFS) and time to progression (TTP) in the overall patient population (n = 75) dichotomized by the median into high (---) and low (—) thymidylate synthase (*TYMS*) gene copy number using FISH probes.

Table 5.2 Hazard ratio (HR) between thymidylate synthase (*TYMS*) gene copy number measured by FISH and progression-free survival (PFS) and time to progression (TTP) in patients treated with capecitabine

TYMS	*PFS*	*TTP*
	HR (P-value)	*HR (P-value)*
Overall population (n = 75)	**1.86 (0.01)**	**1.76 (0.03)**
ER+ (n = 40)	**2.73 (0.01)**	**2.46 (0.02)**
ER− (n = 35)	0.81 (0.55)	0.81 (0.55)
HER2+ (insufficient number)	–	–
HER2− (n = 59)	**2.07 (0.01)**	**1.94 (0.03)**

Table 5.3 Correlation between gene copy number measured by FISH and gene expression measured by DASL in patients treated with capecitabine

Gene (patients)	*Pearson (P-value)*	*Spearman (P-value)*
TYMS (*n* = 57)	**0.26 (0.049)**	0.25 (0.056)
TYMP (*n* = 48)	0.24 (0.1)	0.11 (0.461)
DHFR (*n* = 17)	**−0.64 (0.006)**	-0.41 (0.098)

results suggest that an increased number of *TYMS* gene copies of this gene leads to an increase in its expression and is associated with a decreased benefit from capecitabine therapy. The fact that *TYMS* DASL expression is not associated with outcome may reflect the limitations of RNA extraction from tissue containing many different cell types in addition to cancerous cells, thereby diluting the signal, a situation not encountered in FISH scoring performed exclusively in cancer cells.

Conversely, both PFS and TTP were not significantly different in the patient groups with a high or low *TYMP* gene copy number (Table 5.5 and Figure 5.4) neither was the gene expression correlated with gene copy number (Table 5.3). Interestingly, higher *TYMP* gene expression measured with DASL was associated with significantly decreased HR in the overall population as well as in the *ER*+ and *HER2*– subpopulations, consistent with TYMP's role in activating capecitabine [35] and the fact that it is amplified in tumors by post-transcriptional mechanisms [53] (Table 5.6).

Both PFS and TTP did not correlate with *DHFR* gene copy number whether in the overall patient population or in the different ER and HER2 subgroups (data not shown). Interestingly, a significant inverse correlation was observed between *DHFR* gene copy number and DASL expression (Table 5.3). A higher *DHFR* DASL expression was also associated with a significantly lowered HR for PFS but not TTP in the *ER*+ subgroup (data not shown).

Microarray-based WG-DASL gene expression data were also analyzed using GSEA looking at gene sets grouped either by functional attributes, common transcription factors or chromosomal proximity. The GSEA software (*http://www.broadinstitute.org/gsea/index.jsp*) was used for the analysis and results will be available for publication in the near future.

Conclusions

TYMS

1. Increased *TYMS* gene copy number measured by FISH was associated with reduced capecitabine benefit in the overall population and particularly in the *ER*+ and *HER2*– subpopulations.
2. Protein expression of TYMS was significantly correlated with gene copy number.
3. Although not significant, a similar trend was observed using DASL, suggesting that FISH measured directly in tumor cells is more sensitive than an RNA pool including various cell types.

TYMP

1. *TYMP* gene copy number was not associated with outcome.
2. *TYMP* gene copy number was not significantly correlated with expression, confirming reports that RNA is amplified in tumors by post-transcriptional mechanisms.
3. High *TYMP* DASL expression was significantly associated with increased capecitabine benefit in the overall population (and particularly in the *ER*+ and *HER2*– populations) consistent with its role in activating capecitabine.

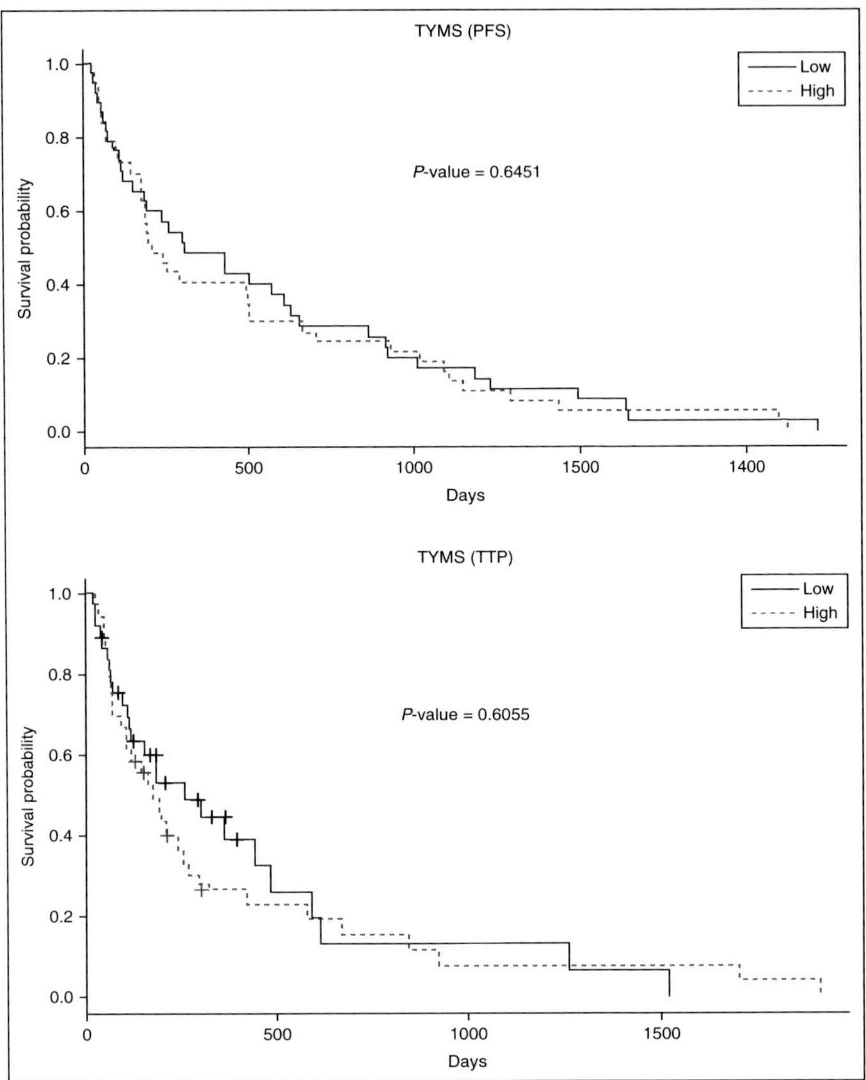

Figure 5.3 Progression-free survival (PFS) and time to progression (TTP) in the overall patient population (n = 73) dichotomized by the median into high (---) and low (—) thymidylate synthase (*TYMS*) gene expression using DASL.

Table 5.4 The impact of thymidylate synthase (*TYMS*) gene expression measured by DASL on progression-free survival (PFS) and time to progression (TTP) in patients treated with capecitabine

TYMS	*PFS*	*TTP*
	HR (P-value)	*HR (P-value)*
Overall population (n = 73)	1.19 (0.16)	1.23 (0.15)
ER+ (n = 40)	1.24 (0.22)	1.46 (0.07)
ER– (n = 33)	1.09 (0.67)	1.05 (0.84)
HER2+ (insufficient number)	–	–
HER2– (n = 60)	1.21 (0.15)	1.17 (0.34)

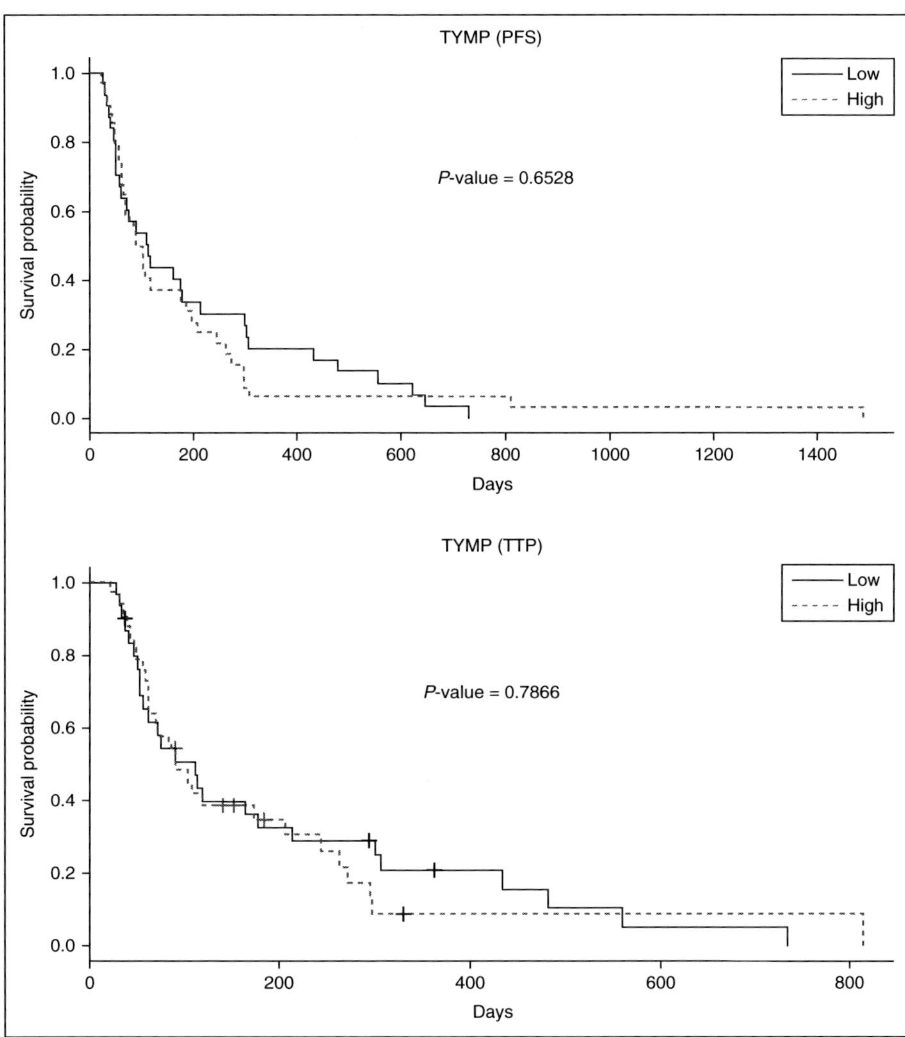

Figure 5.4 Progression-free survival (PFS) and time to progression (TTP) in the overall patient population (*n* = 75) dichotomized by the median into high (---) and low (—) thymidine phosphorylase (*TYMP*) gene copy number using FISH probes.

Table 5.5 The impact of thymidine phosphorylase (*TYMP*) gene copy number measured by FISH on progression-free survival (PFS) and time to progression (TTP) in patients treated with capecitabine

TYMP	*PFS*	*TTP*
	HR (p-value)	*HR (p-value)*
Overall population (*n* = 75)	1.12 (0.65)	1.08 (0.79)
ER+ (*n* = 40)	0.92 (0.83)	0.84 (0.67)
ER− (*n* = 35)	0.82 (0.62)	0.82 (0.65)
HER2+ (insufficient number)	–	–
HER2− (*n* = 59)	1.13 (0.68)	1.08 (0.81)

Table 5.6 The impact of thymidine phosphorylase (*TYMP*) gene expression measured by DASL on progression-free survival (PFS) and time to progression (TTP) in patients treated with capecitabine.

TYMP	*PFS*	*TTP*
	HR (P-value)	*HR (P-value)*
Overall population (n = 75)	**0.17 (0.007)**	0.26 (0.06)
ER+ (n = 41)	**0.1 (0.04)**	0.35 (0.40)
ER− (n = 33)	0.22 (0.07)	0.25 (0.09)
HER2+ (insufficient number)	–	–
HER2− (n = 60)	**0.17 (0.03)**	0.25 (0.12)

DHFR

1. *DHFR* gene copy number was not associated with outcome.
2. *DHFR* gene copy number was inversely correlated with expression.
3. High *DHFR* DASL expression was significantly associated with increased capecitabine benefit in *ER+* patients in line with its role in providing tetrahydrofolate necessary to inactivate the enzyme complex.

A similar correlation between a higher *TYMS* gene copy number and elevated protein expression was associated with decreased benefit from 5-FU adjuvant therapy in colorectal cancer patients [54].

Marker selection rationale for cohort C: vinorelbine

Molecular pharmacology and mechanisms of action

Vinorelbine (Navelbine®) is a semi-synthetic vinca-alkaloid that exhibits antimitotic activity by interfering with the dynamic equilibrium of tubulin [55]. It inhibits tubulin polymerization and preferentially binds to mitotic microtubules causing cell death following a block in mitosis at G2-M [56–58]. Like other vinca-alkaloids it may interfere with amino acid, cyclic adenosine monophosphate (AMP) and glutathione metabolism as well as with calmodulin-dependent Ca-transport or cellular respiration [59]. Vinorelbine is metabolized via deacetylation, hydroxylation, dealkylation and oxidation leading to the generation of many secondary metabolites [60]. Although all of these interactions with intracellular elements represent possible determinants of vinorelbine efficacy, there are relatively few clinical studies addressing this question.

The most obvious and well-studied target of vinorelbine is beta tubulin III (Gene symbol: TUBB3). A recent study has shown that histocultures from lung tumors with high TUBB3 protein levels exhibited greater chemosensitivity to vinorelbine than tumors with lower TUBB3 levels [61]. Conversely, other studies have shown that it is the up-regulation of *TUBB3* which is implicated in drug resistance and not pretreatment levels of *TUBB3* [62].

Vinorelbine was shown to bind with such a high affinity to chromatin that it decreases its melting point and the principal drug binding site is thought to be the globular domain of histones [63, 64]. Modification of histones by methylation or acetylation has been shown to be a key element in gene transcription changes observed in many cancers, including breast [65], and binding of vinorelbine to the histone complex could logically be involved in gene expression involved in the efficacy of this drug.

Our goal was to identify individual genes or gene sets whose expression may affect the efficacy of vinorelbine in breast cancer patients to better individualize therapy.

Results summary for cohort C: vinorelbine

WG-DASL analysis

Forty-three adult female patients with pathologically confirmed breast cancer and locally advanced or metastatic disease were treated with vinorelbine 25 mg/m^2 days 1, 8, 15 of a 28-day cycle. Gene expression was assessed in archival FFPE tissue using the microarray-based WG-DASL assay and correlated with TTP. Using GSEA, gene sets that share a common molecular function, chromosomal location, or regulation were identified in patients classified as having either a short (S) (n = 25) or a long (L) (n = 18) TTP divided by the median (72 days). GSEA software (*http://www.broadinstitute.org/gsea/index.jsp*) was used for the analysis.

Interim GSEA results presented at ASCO 2012 have shown that when genes were grouped according to similar molecular function, 16 out of a set of 43 genes involved in histone binding were enriched in group S (P = 0.002), consistent with higher expression in group S of *HIST3H2BB* and *HIST1H3I*. GSEA analysis of genes grouped according to common transcription factors has shown that 14 out of 47genes were enriched in group S (P = 0.004) including promoter regions that match c-fos serum response element-binding transcription factor and other promoter regions linked to histone expression as well as the cellular membrane pumps *P-gp/MDR1* involved in vinorelbine transport [66].

GSEA analysis of genes grouped according to chromosomal location has shown that in group S genes were enriched on chromosome 11q21 (20 out of 45 genes; P = 0.004) and on chromosome 12p12 (14 out of 22 genes; P = 0.002). These chromosomal regions could represent 'hot spots' where genes are over-expressed following damage or rearrangement of DNA, but further studies are definitively needed in order to unravel the underlying mechanisms.

Conclusions

GSEA suggests that there is an up-regulation of histone-binding genes in patients deriving the least benefit from vinorelbine therapy, which is consonant with the recent discovery of high affinity vinorelbine binding to histones [63, 64]. The role of *P-gp/MDR1* in extracellular transport and resistance to vinorelbine is well known and our finding of an increased transcription factor linked to their expression deserves additional scrutiny as our novel observations on chromosome 11q21 and12p12. DASL expression combined with GSEA highlight gene sets that correlate with clinical outcome and may lead to predictive markers of vinorelbine efficacy. Further confirmatory analysis is needed due to the limitation of small sample size and multiple comparisons.

Marker selection rationale for cohort D: gemcitabine

Molecular pharmacology and mechanisms of action

Gemcitabine (Gemzar®) is a cell cycle-dependent (S-phase-specific) deoxycytidine analogue frequently used in patients with solid tumors; it must first be transported into the cell and phosphorylated to its active triphosphate form. Because gemcitabine is hydrophilic and does not readily cross plasma by passive diffusion in order to gain access to its intracellular targets, it requires the presence of specialized membrane nucleotide transporters [67].

Gemcitabine is taken up into cells via the family of human nucleoside transporters (hNT) including equilibrative (hENT) and concentrative (hCNT) members (Figure 5.5) [68]. hENTs are capable of transporting pyrimidine and purine nucleotides from both outside and inside cells and are widely distributed in human cells. On the other hand, hCNTs can transport pyrimidines and purines across the cellular membrane against a concentration gradient and generally have a higher affinity for transport of nucleotides than hENTs (i.e. hCNT1 has a tenfold higher affinity for gemcitabine than hENT1) [67].

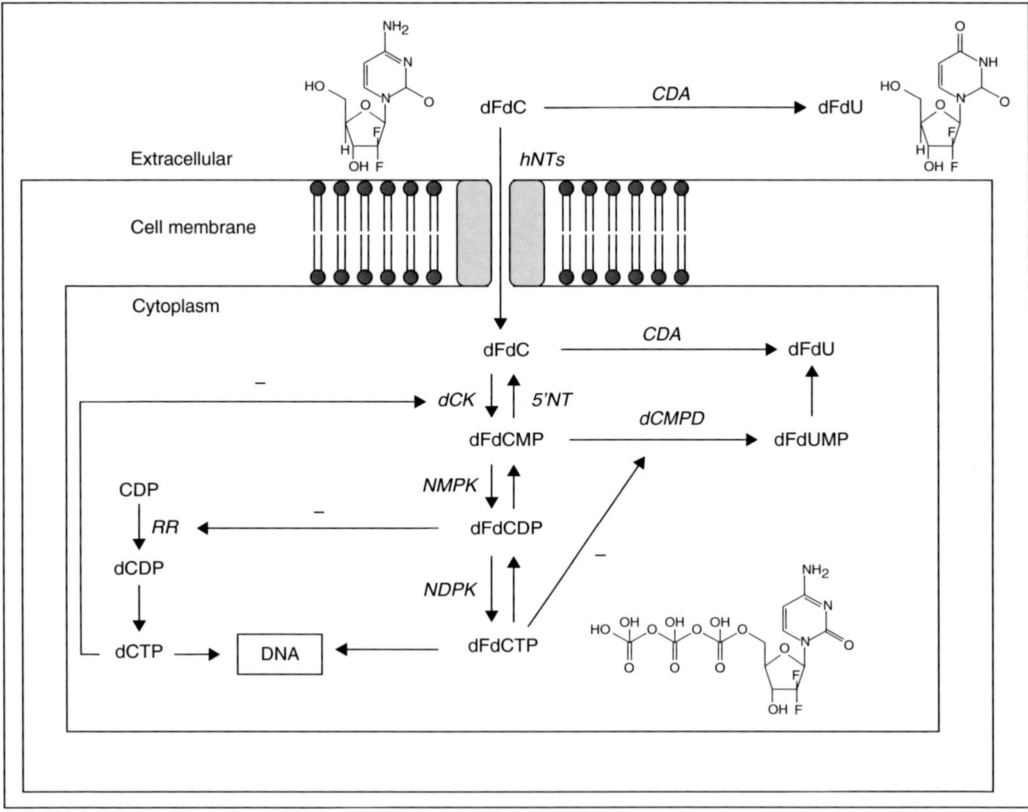

Figure 5.5 Pathway of gemcitabine metabolism and catabolism.

Abbreviations: 5′-NT, 5′-nucleotidase; CDA, cytidine deaminase; CDP, cytidine diphosphate; dCDP, deoxycytidine diphosphate; dCK, deoxycytidine kinase; dCMPD, deoxycytidylate deaminase; dCTP, deoxycytidine triphosphate; dFdC, 2′,2′-difluorodeoxycytidine; dFdCDP, dFdC diphosphate; dFdCMP, dFdC monophosphate; dFdCTP, dFdC triphosphate; dFdU, 2′,2′-difluorodeoxyuridine; dFdUMP, 2′,2′-difluorodeoxyuridine monophosphate; hNTs, human nucleoside transporters; RR, ribonucleotide reductase.

hENT1 is known as member 1 of the solute carrier family 29 (gene abbreviation: *SLC29A1*). hCNT2 is officially known as member 2 of the solute carrier family 28 (gene abbreviation: *SLC28A2*).

Phosphorylation of gemcitabine by deoxycytidine kinase (dCK) is the first and rate-limiting step of the formation of its active form, fluorodeoxycytidine monophosphate (dFdCMP) before being transformed into its main active metabolite 2′-2′-difluorodeoxycytidine triphosphate (dFdCTP), which is incorporated into DNA and inhibits DNA synthesis [68].

Results summary for gemcitabine

Data are being compiled and will include IHC analysis of ENT, DCK and CNT as well as expression analysis using either DASL or qRT-PCR for *ENT*, *DCK*, *CNT* and *RRM1* (Table 5.1). These data will allow the assessment of changes at both the mRNA and protein levels and the correlation of these with benefits from gemcitabine chemotherapy. GSEA will also be performed and should hopefully bring new insights into the tumor characteristics that have an impact on clinical outcome of gemcitabine chemotherapy.

SUMMARY

Marker discovery and development is a complex, time-consuming and expensive enterprise, which can be simplified greatly by the use of good quality archival specimens. Nevertheless, our interim data are promising and clearly show that, although pinpointing a particular phenotype associated with a clinical outcome is challenging, new integrated methods are available and hold the promise of better targeted classical chemotherapy.

Acknowledgements

Department of Defense Award through the Breast Cancer Research Program W81XWH-04-1-0468 "Center of Excellence for Individualization of Therapy for Breast Cancer". The authors wish to thank the following colleagues for their assistance in the preparation and writing of this chapter: J. Jeong, T. Breen, B. Young, K. Vang Nielsen, K. Adamowicz, J. Zok, W. Rogowski, M. Litwiniuk, S. Debska, M. Jaworska, M. Foszczynska-Kloda, M. Kulma-Kreft, K. Zabkowska, J. Jassem, S. Edgerton and B. R. Smith.

REFERENCES

1. Oostendorp LJ, Stalmeier PF, Donders AR, van der Graaf WT, Ottevanger PB. Efficacy and safety of palliative chemotherapy for patients with advanced breast cancer pretreated with anthracyclines and taxanes: a systematic review. *Lancet Oncol* 2011; 12:1053–1061.
2. Beslija S, Bonneterre J, Burstein HJ *et al*. Third consensus on medical treatment of metastatic breast cancer. *Ann Oncol* 2009; 20:1771–1785.
3. Cardoso F, Fallowfield L, Costa A, Castiglione M, Senkus E. Locally recurrent or metastatic breast cancer: ESMO Clinical Practice Guidelines for diagnosis, treatment and follow-up. *Ann Oncol* 2011; 22(suppl 6):vi25–vi30.
4. Early Breast Cancer Trialists' Collaborative Group (EBCTCG). Effects of chemotherapy and hormonal therapy for early breast cancer on recurrence and 15-year survival: an overview of the randomised trials. *Lancet* 2005; 365:1687–1717.
5. Sauter G, Lee J, Bartlett JM, Slamon DJ, Press MF. Guidelines for human epidermal growth factor receptor 2 testing: biologic and methodologic considerations. *J Clin Oncol* 2009; 27:1323–1333.
6. Mackey JR, Jennings LL, Clarke ML *et al*. Immunohistochemical variation of human equilibrative nucleoside transporter 1 protein in primary breast cancers. *Clin Cancer Res* 2002; 8:110–116.
7. Hatzis P, Al Madhoon AS, Jullig M, Petrakis TG, Eriksson S, Talianidis I. The intracellular localization of deoxycytidine kinase. *J Biol Chem* 1998; 273:30239–30243.
8. de Jonge ME, Huitema AD, Rodenhuis S, Beijnen JH. Clinical pharmacokinetics of cyclophosphamide. *Clin Pharmacokinet* 2005; 44:1135–1164.
9. Huitema AD, Smits KD, Mathot RA, Schellens JH, Rodenhuis S, Beijnen JH. The clinical pharmacology of alkylating agents in high-dose chemotherapy. *Anticancer Drugs* 2000; 11:515–533.
10. Bunting KD, Townsend AJ. De novo expression of transfected human class 1 aldehyde dehydrogenase (ALDH) causes resistance to oxazaphosphorine anti-cancer alkylating agents in hamster V79 cell lines. Elevated class 1 ALDH activity is closely correlated with reduction in DNA interstrand cross-linking and lethality. *J Biol Chem* 1996; 271:11884–11890.
11. DeMichele A, Aplenc R, Botbyl J *et al*. Drug-metabolizing enzyme polymorphisms predict clinical outcome in a node-positive breast cancer cohort. *J Clin Oncol* 2005; 23:5552–5559.
12. DeMichele A, Gimotty P, Botbyl J *et al*. In response to "Drug metabolizing enzyme polymorphisms predict clinical outcome in a node-positive breast cancer cohort". *J Clin Oncol* 2007; 25:5675–5677.

13. Su HI, Sammel MD, Velders L *et al*. Association of cyclophosphamide drug-metabolizing enzyme polymorphisms and chemotherapy-related ovarian failure in breast cancer survivors. *Fertil Steril* 2010; 94:645–654.
14. Gor PP, Su HI, Gray RJ *et al*. Cyclophosphamide-metabolizing enzyme polymorphisms and survival outcomes after adjuvant chemotherapy for node-positive breast cancer: a retrospective cohort study. *Breast Cancer Res* 2010; 12:R26.
15. Moreb JS. Aldehyde dehydrogenase as a marker for stem cells. *Curr Stem Cell Res Ther* 2008; 3:237–246.
16. Sladek NE, Kollander R, Sreerama L, Kiang DT. Cellular levels of aldehyde dehydrogenases (ALDH1A1 and ALDH3A1) as predictors of therapeutic responses to cyclophosphamide-based chemotherapy of breast cancer: a retrospective study. Rational individualization of oxazaphosphorine-based cancer chemotherapeutic regimens. *Cancer Chemother Pharmacol* 2002; 49:309–321.
17. Bunting KD, Lindahl R, Townsend AJ. Oxazaphosphorine-specific resistance in human MCF-7 breast carcinoma cell lines expressing transfected rat class 3 aldehyde dehydrogenase. *J Biol Chem* 1994; 269:23197–23203.
18. Ekhart C, Doodeman VD, Rodenhuis S, Smits PH, Beijnen JH, Huitema AD. Influence of polymorphisms of drug metabolizing enzymes (CYP2B6, CYP2C9, CYP2C19, CYP3A4, CYP3A5, GSTA1, GSTP1, ALDH1A1 and ALDH3A1) on the pharmacokinetics of cyclophosphamide and 4-hydroxycyclophosphamide. *Pharmacogenet Genomics* 2008; 18:515–523.
19. Levi BP, Yilmaz OH, Duester G, Morrison SJ. Aldehyde dehydrogenase 1a1 is dispensable for stem cell function in the mouse hematopoietic and nervous systems. *Blood* 2008; 113(8):1670–1680.
20. Sreerama L, Sladek NE. Cellular levels of class 1 and class 3 aldehyde dehydrogenases and certain other drug-metabolizing enzymes in human breast malignancies. *Clin Cancer Res* 1997; 3:1901–1914.
21. Pritchard KI, Messersmith H, Elavathil L, Trudeau M, O'Malley F, Dhesy-Thind B. HER-2 and topoisomerase II as predictors of response to chemotherapy. *J Clin Oncol* 2008; 26:736–744.
22. Järvinen TA, Tanner M, Barlund M, Borg A, Isola J. Characterization of topoisomerase II alpha gene amplification and deletion in breast cancer. *Genes Chromosomes Cancer* 1999; 26:142–150.
23. Järvinen TA, Tanner M, Rantanen V *et al*. Amplification and deletion of topoisomerase IIalpha associate with ErbB-2 amplification and affect sensitivity to topoisomerase II inhibitor doxorubicin in breast cancer. *Am J Pathol* 2000; 156:839–847.
24. Zaczek A, Markiewicz A, Jaskiewicz J *et al*. Clinical evaluation of developed PCR-based method with hydrolysis probes for TOP2A copy number evaluation in breast cancer samples. *Clin Biochem* 2010; 43:891–898.
25. Corzo C, Bellosillo B, Corominas JM *et al*. Does polysomy of chromosome 17 have a role in ERBB2 and topoisomerase IIalpha expression? Gene, mRNA and protein expression: a comprehensive analysis. *Tumour Biol* 2007; 28:221–228.
26. Moretti E, Oakman C, Di Leo A. Predicting anthracycline benefit: have we made any progress? *Curr Opin Oncol* 2009; 21:507–515.
27. Oakman C, Moretti E, Galardi F, Santarpia L, Di Leo A. The role of topoisomerase IIalpha and HER-2 in predicting sensitivity to anthracyclines in breast cancer patients. *Cancer Treat Rev* 2009; 35:662–667.
28. Hicks DG, Yoder BJ, Pettay J *et al*. The incidence of topoisomerase II-alpha genomic alterations in adenocarcinoma of the breast and their relationship to human epidermal growth factor receptor-2 gene amplification: a fluorescence in situ hybridization study. *Hum Pathol* 2005; 36:348–356.
29. Orlando L, Del Curto B, Gandini S *et al*. Topoisomerase IIalpha gene status and prediction of pathological complete remission after anthracycline-based neoadjuvant chemotherapy in endocrine non-responsive Her2/neu-positive breast cancer. *Breast* 2008; 17:506–511.
30. Zaczek AJ, Markiewicz A, Seroczynska B *et al*. Prognostic significance of TOP2A gene dosage in HER-2-negative breast cancer. *Oncologist* 2012: Sept 14 [Epub ahead of print].
31. Glynn RW, Miller N, Kerin MJ. 17q12–21 – the pursuit of targeted therapy in breast cancer. *Cancer Treat Rev* 2010; 36:224–229.
32. Nielsen KV, Müller S, Møller S *et al*. Aberrations of ERBB2 and TOP2A genes in breast cancer. *Mol Oncol* 2010; 4:161–168.
33. Desmedt C, Di Leo A, de Azambuja E *et al*. Multifactorial approach to predicting resistance to anthracyclines. *J Clin Oncol* 2011; 29:1578–1586.
34. García-Bilbao A, Rubén Armañanzas R, Ispizua Z *et al*. Identification of a biomarker panel for colorectal cancer diagnosis. *BMC Cancer* 2012; 12:43 (doi:10.1186/1471–2407–12–43).

35. Miwa M, Ura M, Nishida M *et al.* Design of a novel oral fluoropyrimidine carbamate, capecitabine, which generates 5-fluorouracil selectively in tumours by enzymes concentrated in human liver and cancer tissue. *Eur J Cancer* 1998; 34:1274–1281.
36. Takebayashi Y, Yamada K, Miyadera K *et al.* The activity and expression of thymidine phosphorylase in human solid tumours. *Eur J Cancer* 1996; 32A:1227–1232.
37. Kobayashi M, Sugimoto T, Okabayashi T *et al.* Localization of thymidine phosphorylase in breast cancer tissue. *Med Mol Morphol* 2005; 38:112–117.
38. Walko CM, Lindley C. Capecitabine: a review. *Clin Ther* 2005; 27:23–44.
39. Peters GJ, van der Wilt CL, van Triest B *et al.* Thymidylate synthase and drug resistance. *Eur J Cancer* 1995; 31A:1299–1305.
40. Houghton JA, Schmidt C, Houghton PJ. The effect of derivatives of folic acid on the fluorodeoxyuridylate-thymidylate synthetase covalent complex in human colon xenografts. *Eur J Cancer Clin Oncol* 1982; 18:347–354.
41. Houghton JA, Houghton PJ. Elucidation of pathways of 5-fluorouracil metabolism in xenografts of human colorectal adenocarcinoma. *Eur J Cancer Clin Oncol* 1983; 19:807–815.
42. Capiaux GM, Budak-Alpdogan T, Takebe N *et al.* Retroviral transduction of a mutant dihydrofolate reductase-thymidylate synthase fusion gene into murine marrow cells confers resistance to both methotrexate and 5-fluorouracil. *Hum Gene Ther* 2003; 14:435–446.
43. Will CL, Dolnick BJ. 5-Fluorouracil inhibits dihydrofolate reductase precursor mRNA processing and/or nuclear mRNA stability in methotrexate-resistant KB cells. *J Biol Chem* 1989; 264:21413–21421.
44. Johnson MR, Wang K, Tillmanns S, Albin N, Diasio RB. Structural organization of the human dihydropyrimidine dehydrogenase gene. *Cancer Res* 1997; 57:1660–1663.
45. Lee A, Ezzeldin H, Fourie J, Diasio R. Dihydropyrimidine dehydrogenase deficiency: impact of pharmacogenetics on 5-fluorouracil therapy. *Clin Adv Hematol Oncol* 2004; 2:527–532.
46. Lu Z, Zhang R, Diasio RB. Dihydropyrimidine dehydrogenase activity in human peripheral blood mononuclear cells and liver: population characteristics, newly identified deficient patients, and clinical implication in 5-fluorouracil chemotherapy. *Cancer Res* 1993; 53:5433–5438.
47. Kornmann M, Schwabe W, Sander S *et al.* Thymidylate synthase and dihydropyrimidine dehydrogenase mRNA expression levels: predictors for survival in colorectal cancer patients receiving adjuvant 5-fluorouracil. *Clin Cancer Res* 2003; 9:4116–4124.
48. Kobunai T, Ooyama A, Sasaki S *et al.* Changes to the dihydropyrimidine dehydrogenase gene copy number influence the susceptibility of cancers to 5-FU-based drugs: Data mining of the NCI-DTP data sets and validation with human tumour xenografts. *Eur J Cancer* 2007; 43:791–798.
49. Ishikawa T, Sekiguchi F, Fukase Y, Sawada N, Ishitsuka H. Positive correlation between the efficacy of capecitabine and doxifluridine and the ratio of thymidine phosphorylase to dihydropyrimidine dehydrogenase activities in tumors in human cancer xenografts. *Cancer Res* 1998; 58:685–690.
50. Honda J, Sasa M, Moriya T *et al.* Thymidine phosphorylase and dihydropyrimidine dehydrogenase are predictive factors of therapeutic efficacy of capecitabine monotherapy for breast cancer – preliminary results. *J Med Invest* 2008; 55:54–60.
51. Kakimoto M, Uetake H, Osanai T *et al.* Thymidylate synthase and dihydropyrimidine dehydrogenase gene expression in breast cancer predicts 5-FU sensitivity by a histocultural drug sensitivity test. *Cancer Lett* 2005; 223:103–111.
52. Tominaga T, Toi M, Ohashi Y, Abe O. Prognostic and predictive value of thymidine phosphorylase activity in early-stage breast cancer patients. *Clin Breast Cancer* 2002; 3:55–64.
53. Toi M, Atiqur RM, Bando H, Chow LW. Thymidine phosphorylase (platelet-derived endothelial-cell growth factor) in cancer biology and treatment. *Lancet Oncol* 2005; 6:158–166.
54. Jensen SA, Vainer B, Witton CJ, Jorgensen JT, Sorensen JB. Prognostic significance of numeric aberrations of genes for thymidylate synthase, thymidine phosphorylase and dihydrofolate reductase in colorectal cancer. *Acta Oncol* 2008; 47:1054–1061.
55. Lobert S, Vulevic B, Correia JJ. Interaction of vinca alkaloids with tubulin: a comparison of vinblastine, vincristine, and vinorelbine. *Biochemistry* 1996; 35:6806–6814.
56. Binet S, Fellous A, Lataste H, Krikorian A, Couzinier JP, Meininger V. In situ analysis of the action of Navelbine on various types of microtubules using immunofluorescence. *Semin Oncol* 1989; 16:5–8.
57. Fellous A, Ohayon R, Vacassin T *et al.* Biochemical effects of Navelbine on tubulin and associated proteins. *Semin Oncol* 1989; 16:9–14.

58. Goa KL, Faulds D. Vinorelbine. A review of its pharmacological properties and clinical use in cancer chemotherapy. *Drugs Aging* 1994; 5:200–234.
59. Galano G, Caputo M, Tecce MF, Capasso A. Efficacy and tolerability of vinorelbine in the cancer therapy. *Curr Drug Saf* 2011; 6:185–193.
60. de Graeve J, van Heugen JC, Zorza G, Fahy J, Puozzo C. Metabolism pathway of vinorelbine (Navelbine) in human: Characterisation of the metabolites by HPLC-MS/MS. *J Pharm Biomed Anal* 2008; 47:47–58.
61. Hirai Y, Yoshimasu T, Oura S *et al.* Is class III beta-tubulin a true predictive marker of sensitivity to vinorelbine in non-small cell lung cancer? Chemosensitivity data evidence. *Anticancer Res* 2011; 31:999–1005.
62. Saussede-Aim J, Matera EL, Herveau S, Rouault JP, Ferlini C, Dumontet C. Vinorelbine induces beta3-tubulin gene expression through an AP-1 Site. *Anticancer Res* 2009; 29:3003–3009.
63. Rabbani-Chadegani A, Chamani E, Hajihassan Z. The effect of vinca alkaloid anticancer drug, vinorelbine, on chromatin and histone proteins in solution. *Eur J Pharmacol* 2009; 613:34–38.
64. Rabbani-Chadegani A, Keyvani-Ghamsari S, Zarkar N. Spectroscopic studies of dactinomycin and vinorelbine binding to deoxyribonucleic acid and chromatin. *Spectrochim Acta A Mol Biomol Spectrosc* 2011; 84:62–67.
65. Stratmann A, Haendler B. Histone demethylation and steroid receptor function in cancer. *Mol Cell Endocrinol* 2012; 348:12–20.
66. Wong M, Balleine RL, Blair EY *et al.* Predictors of vinorelbine pharmacokinetics and pharmacodynamics in patients with cancer. *J Clin Oncol* 2006; 24:2448–2455.
67. Mackey JR, Mani RS, Selner M *et al.* Functional nucleoside transporters are required for gemcitabine influx and manifestation of toxicity in cancer cell lines. *Cancer Res* 1998; 58:4349–4357.
68. Veltkamp SA, Beijnen JH, Schellens JH. Prolonged versus standard gemcitabine infusion: translation of molecular pharmacology to new treatment strategy. *Oncologist* 2008; 13:261–276.

6

Antiangiogenic therapy for breast cancer

G. W. Sledge Jr.

INTRODUCTION

Antiangiogenic therapy for breast cancer first burst onto the scene in 2005 with the reporting of results from the US Intergroup trial E2100, which demonstrated highly statistical improvement (in both relative and absolute terms) in progression-free survival (PFS) for front-line metastatic breast cancer. Subsequent phase III trials with bevacizumab reported statistically significant (but inferior to E2100's) PFS, and analysis of all three trials (both individually and collectively) showed no overall survival benefit for bevacizumab. This failure to demonstrate a survival benefit, combined with the variable PFS results and real toxicity of bevacizumab, led to the US Food and Drug Administration's withdrawal of bevacizumab's indication in metastatic breast cancer.

The withdrawal of bevacizumab's indication in metastatic breast cancer suggests that it is time to re-evaluate the role, not just of bevacizumab, but also of antiangiogenic therapy as a whole, as targeted therapy for breast cancer. Several questions are worth addressing:

1. What is the biologic rationale for antiangiogenic therapy in metastatic breast cancer?
2. What data suggest clinical benefit (or lack thereof) of antiangiogenic therapy for breast cancer?
3. Does antiangiogenic therapy represent targeted therapy for breast cancer, and if not can it evolve towards targeted therapy?
4. What are the future prospects for antiangiogenic therapy in breast cancer?

BIOLOGIC RATIONALE FOR ANTIANGIOGENIC THERAPY IN BREAST CANCER

There are several reasons to believe that antiangiogenic therapy might prove beneficial in breast cancer. First, data from as long ago as the early 1990s suggested that the prognosis of patients with early stage breast cancer is related to measures of blood vessel formation in general (e.g. microvessel density in human breast cancers [1]) and to specific proangiogenic growth factors in particular. The most robust datasets exist for vascular endothelial growth factor (VEGF) (reviewed in [2]). Increased VEGF content is associated with impaired clinical outcome (i.e. VEGF is prognostic in early breast cancer) as well as resistance to both hormonal therapy and chemotherapy (i.e. VEGF is predictive of therapeutic response to standard breast cancer therapies) [2].

George W. Sledge, Jr., MD, Professor, Department of Medicine; Chief, Division of Oncology, Stanford University School of Medicine, Palo Alto, California, USA.

Angiogenesis is a hallmark of breast carcinogenesis, with both increased microvessel density and increased VEGF production occurring at the transition from atypical hyperplasia to in situ carcinoma [3, 4]. In invasive breast cancer, angiogenesis and VEGF production are most prominent in the most inherently aggressive breast cancers, correlating with aggressive intrinsic subtypes (HER2-positive and triple negative breast cancers) and poor histologic differentiation [5, 6].

In multiple preclinical models of breast cancer, antiangiogenic therapy attacking multiple points of the angiogenic cascade results in diminished tumor growth, and the combination of anti-VEGF therapy with other breast cancer therapies (including both chemotherapy and HER2-targeted therapy) results in additive or synergistic antitumor effects [5–7].

Antiangiogenic therapy therefore represented a biologically rational approach to breast cancer therapy. In retrospect, preclinical model systems, and some clinical data, pointed to potential problems in its application to breast cancer patients. First, early analyses of primary breast cancer tumors suggested that the invocation of multiple proangiogenic molecules in the same tumor was a common occurrence, suggesting the existence of compensatory mechanisms from the outset of disease diagnosis [8]. Secondly, preclinical models suggested the potential for rapid regrowth of endothelial cells following cessation of antiangiogenic therapy, with the associated threat of rapid blood vessel and tumor regrowth [9]. Third, murine models suggested that VEGF blockade in particular was associated with the rapid emergence of host-derived compensatory mechanisms, with the production of both cytokines and marrow-derived endothelial progenitor cells [10, 11]. Finally, relatively little attention was paid to combinations of antiangiogenic therapies with standard breast cancer therapies (particularly chemotherapy type) in preclinical models. This tendency to assume that all cancers would respond similarly to antiangiogenic therapies is a common failing across tumor types.

ANTIANGIOGENIC THERAPY IN THE CLINIC: PHASE III TRIAL EXPERIENCE

The anti-VEGF ligand monoclonal antibody was the first therapeutic agent to be comprehensively evaluated in a clinical setting. Following initial phase I safety trials, a phase II monotherapy trial was performed in patients with advanced metastatic breast cancer [12]. This trial demonstrated modest but real therapeutic activity in metastatic breast cancer, and led to the development of phase III trials in refractory and front-line metastatic breast cancer.

The first of these, the 2119 trial, randomized patients with taxane-refractory metastatic breast cancer to receive capecitabine with or without bevacizumab. This trial failed to demonstrate a benefit for its primary endpoint of PFS, though it did demonstrate a doubling in overall response rate [13]. A subsequent trial (the RIBBON-2 trial) examined a broader range of second-line treatments, and allowed physicians to choose between capecitabine, a taxane (paclitaxel, nab-paclitaxel, or docetaxel), gemcitabine, or vinorelbine, administered with either bevacizumab or a placebo. Only the capecitabine population was powered to address benefit with an individual drug. This trial was positive in its primary PFS endpoint for the overall group (5.1 vs. 7.2 months; $P = 0.0072$), but did not result in an improvement in overall survival [14].

In the subsequently reported front-line metastatic US Breast Cancer Intergroup trial E2100 patients were randomized to receive paclitaxel on a weekly basis with or without bevacizumab. As with the previous capecitabine trial, PFS was the primary endpoint. In contrast to that trial, however, the addition of bevacizumab to front-line paclitaxel resulted in a doubling in PFS from 5.9 to 11.8 months, at the time the largest improvement in PFS ever seen in a metastatic breast cancer trial. Forrest plot analyses of E2100 failed to demonstrate any subset with greater or lesser benefit with anti-VEGF therapy. Based upon these results, the US FDA gave accelerated approval to bevacizumab in February of 2008, with subsequent approval by European regulatory authorities.

Treatment-related toxicity in E2100, and in subsequent trials, was consistent with the known side effects of anti-VEGF therapy seen in all trials. These include the predominantly mechanistic side effects of hypertension, proteinuria, arterial and venous thromboembolic effects, migraine-like headaches, bleeding or hemorrhage (particularly nosebleeds), congestive heart failure and gastrointestinal perforation. Of these, hypertension is the most common grade 3/4 side effect, but is in general readily manageable with standard antihypertensive agents.

Subsequent phase III trials with bevacizumab in front-line metastatic breast cancer included the AVADO [15] and RIBBON-1 [16] trials. Similarly to E2100, these trials were performed in patients with HER2-negative disease. The AVADO trial randomized patients to receive docetaxel with or without bevacizumab, whereas the RIBBON-1 trial randomized patients to receive one of a number of non-paclitaxel chemotherapeutics (chosen by the physician) with or without bevacizumab. These trials, like the original E2100 trial, demonstrated statistically significant improvements in PFS, and a lack of a suggestion of any preferential clinically applicable subset for benefit. These results were therefore supportive of the use of bevacizumab from a proof-of-concept standpoint.

Unfortunately, and also like E2100, these trials failed to demonstrate an overall survival benefit. And in contrast to the E2100 trial, AVADO and RIBBON-1 showed inferior PFS results, with a median of 0.7 and 2.9 months improvement compared to their chemotherapy comparator. Based on these results, the US FDA convened a meeting of its Oncology Drug Advisory Committee, which recommended removal of bevacizumab's label, beginning a process that concluded with the label's removal by the commissioner of the FDA in November 2011. The basis for this removal was the perception that bevacizumab's PFS benefits, viewed *in toto*, were outweighed by its toxicities in the absence of an overall survival benefit.

Numerous other anti-VEGF therapies were evaluated subsequent to bevacizumab in metastatic breast cancer. Sunitinib, the best studied of these, will serve as a surrogate for small molecule receptor tyrosine kinase inhibitors of VEGF receptors (particularly VEGFR-2). Sunitinib inhibits VEGFR-2, PDGF, c-Kit and (to a lesser degree) several other receptor tyrosine kinases at clinically achievable doses. Several sunitinib-based phase III trials in metastatic breast cancer have been performed. Perhaps the most important was a first-line trial randomizing patients to receive either sunitinib plus paclitaxel or bevacizumab plus paclitaxel (the latter in the dose and schedule employed in the E2100 trial) [17]. This trial was terminated because of futility. Median PFS was shorter with sunitinib–paclitaxel (7.4 vs. 9.2 months; hazard ratio [HR] 1.63; [95% confidence interval (CI), 1.18–2.25]; 1-sided P = 0.999), and the bevacizumab-containing arm was better tolerated, with fewer grade 3/4 neutropenic events. A companion phase III trial randomized front-line patients to receive docetaxel alone or in combination with sunitinib as front-line therapy. Similar to the paclitaxel-based trial, this study failed to demonstrate either PFS or overall survival benefit [18].

Sunitinib has been compared to capecitabine in a phase III trial in taxane-refractory metastatic breast cancer. In this trial, sunitinib underperformed capecitabine with regard to PFS, and the study was halted for futility [19]. This study strongly suggests the inefficacy of single-agent antiangiogenic therapy in breast cancer. Collectively, the phase III sunitinib trials demonstrate a lack of clinical benefit of this agent in breast cancer.

Numerous other anti-VEGF targeting agents have entered clinical trials, but will not be discussed here as none have demonstrated either PFS or overall survival benefit in metastatic breast cancer.

HER2-positive breast cancer represents a special area of interest for anti-VEGF therapy in breast cancer. HER2-positive breast cancers produce increased amounts of VEGF ligand, both in the laboratory and the clinic, and preclinical models of HER2-positive breast cancer suggest therapeutic synergy of HER2-targeting and VEGF-targeting therapeutics. Initial clinical trial results combining trastuzumab and bevacizumab also suggested increased combinatorial activity.

These results naturally led to the development of phase III trials of combination anti-HER2 and anti-VEGF therapy in multiple disease settings. The recently reported AVEREL trial randomized patients receiving front-line docetaxel and trastuzumab for HER2-positive disease to either a placebo or to bevacizumab. As reported at the 2011 San Antonio Breast Cancer Symposium, the addition of bevacizumab to trastuzumab-based therapy in this setting resulted in a 2.5-month median improvement in PFS but – as in HER2-negative metastatic breast cancer – no improvement in overall survival.

Anti-VEGF therapy has also been combined with hormonal therapy in the setting of metastatic breast cancer, with trials being performed in both the United States and Europe. The first of these to be presented (at the 2012 San Antonio Breast Cancer Symposium), the LEA trial, randomized front-line estrogen receptor-positive metastatic breast cancer patients to receive either hormonal therapy alone (with letrozole or fulvestrant) or in combination with bevacizumab 15 mg/kg every 3 weeks. The addition of anti-VEGF therapy failed to improve either progression-free or overall survival, suggesting a lack of any obvious synergies between the two [20].

In summary, then, there is clear proof-of-concept evidence suggesting that bevacizumab perturbs the natural history of metastatic breast cancer in the front-line setting, whether in ER-positive, triple-negative, or HER2-positive disease, with routine increases in these trials' primary endpoint of PFS. Despite this, these same trials consistently fail to demonstrate an overall survival benefit.

IS ANTI-VEGF THERAPY A TARGETED THERAPY FOR METASTATIC BREAST CANCER?

There are many potential explanations, none of which are easily amenable to proof and all of which may apply. Patients in front-line metastatic breast cancer spend only a small proportion of their metastatic life on bevacizumab, and the multiple available lines of subsequent chemotherapy might dilute any overall survival benefit [21]. Similarly, as all of the trials performed discontinued bevacizumab at disease progression, removal of VEGF inhibition might result in the rebound effect seen in preclinical models [9]. Recent work suggests that anti-VEGF therapy increases the breast cancer stem cell population in preclinical models [22]. The use of possibly inadequate durations of chemotherapy (such as occurred with docetaxel in the AVADO trial) may have reduced PFS in these trials and thereby decreased the likelihood of obtaining an overall survival benefit.

One possible explanation has intrigued investigators hoping to reverse the FDA's negative verdict. Anti-VEGF therapy is not clearly targeted therapy, and the lack of a clearly targetable patient population might have resulted in results inferior to those that might have been obtained with an appropriate biomarker of response.

At first glance the claim that anti-VEGF is not targeted therapy might seem absurd: the monoclonal antibody has a highly specific affinity for the VEGF ligand. Yet the reality is that we are not yet capable of demonstrating that measurement of the VEGF ligand (in the case of bevacizumab), or of other factors in tumor or serum, predict clinical outcome. We cannot identify a specific population benefitting from therapy, and therefore lack a means of limiting therapy.

Pegram *et al.* examined the effects of this failure in simulation models, demonstrating that lack of a surrogate biomarker of response hugely decreases the statistical power of a phase III trial to demonstrate clinical benefit [23]. Might this explain the negative overall survival results seen in the metastatic bevacizumab trials, at least in part?

There have been several attempts to identify a group of patients receiving therapeutic benefit with bevacizumab, as recently discussed by Schneider and Sledge [24]. Measures of circulating VEGF and VEGF receptors have shown variable results, as have measures of tumor VEGF and VEGF receptors. Schneider *et al.*, using tumor samples from the E2100 trial, demonstrated a statistically significant relation between VEGF single nucleotide polymorphisms and overall survival in patients receiving bevacizumab, though not (curiously) a relation with the trial's primary endpoint of PFS [25]. The search for appropriate biomarkers of benefit continues with ongoing genomic analyses of E2100 and other phase III trials.

FUTURE PROSPECTS: THE ADJUVANT AND NEOADJUVANT SETTING

Anti-VEGF therapies continue to be studied, and the final verdict on this class of agents has not yet been handed down. Trials of anti-VEGF therapy in both HER2-negative and HER2-positive early stage breast cancer have finished accrual and are awaiting sufficient follow-up and adequate numbers of events for analysis. The E5103 North American Breast Cancer Intergroup trial randomized HER2-negative patients to receive either a backbone chemotherapy regimen of doxorubicin and cyclophosphamide followed by weekly paclitaxel alone or with bevacizumab, with a primary endpoint of disease-free survival.

Similarly, the BETH trial randomizes HER2-positive early stage patients to receive chemotherapy and trastuzumab, either alone or in combination with bevacizumab. As with the E5103 trial, disease-free survival is the primary endpoint of this trial.

Both trials have made significant efforts to obtain paraffin-embedded tumor tissues as well as blood samples for biomarker analysis, and it is hoped that such samples will prove useful in developing biomarkers of therapeutic benefit for anti-VEGF therapy. The E5103 trial in particular has already demonstrated the benefit of this approach. VEGF single nucleotide polymorphism (SNP) analysis of E5103 DNA samples has confirmed an earlier observation of a correlation of VEGF SNPs with the development of hypertension. Additional genome-wide association studies (GWAS) have been performed on DNA obtained from E5103 patients and should provide useful information for years to come.

Preoperative, or neoadjuvant, trials frequently allow physicians to get a first look at the outcomes of adjuvant trials. Two randomized phase III neoadjuvant trials have recently been reported [26, 27]. Bear *et al.* reported the results of a trial randomizing women to receive one of several chemotherapy regimens, with a secondary randomization to either receive or not receive bevacizumab administered with chemotherapy. Patients receiving bevacizumab had a higher overall pathologic complete response (pCR) rate (34.5% vs. 28.2%; $P = 0.02$) [27]. In the study by von Minckwitz *et al.* of the German Breast Group, pCR rate was also increased by bevacizumab (18.4% vs. 14.9%; $P = 0.04$) [26]. Confusingly, subset analyses in the two studies provided differing benefit signals based on intrinsic subtype. Whether these modest improvements in pCR rates in the adjuvant setting will translate to significant clinical benefit remains to be seen.

Preclinical modeling has raised concerns over the role of anti-VEGF therapy in the micrometastatic setting. Ebos *et al.* have reported increased growth in an adjuvant setting in response to the small molecule receptor tyrosine kinase inhibitor sunitinib [28], though the applicability of such models to early stage breast cancer is uncertain [29].

CONCLUSION

Antiangiogenic therapy continues to attract the attention and interest of investigators in both lab and clinic, despite the disappointments associated with clinical trials of anti-VEGF therapies in breast cancer. The biologic rationale underlying antiangiogenic therapy remains a compelling one: new blood vessel formation, after all, is a hallmark of cancer in general and breast cancer in particular. The biologic plausibility of this hypothesis has been confirmed rather that denied by phase III trials in the metastatic disease setting, where bevacizumab has consistently been associated with improvements in median PFS.

At the same time, antiangiogenic therapy has clearly been punished for its inability to produce a reproducible, biologically plausible biomarker of response. If antiangiogenic therapy is to join the ranks of HER2- and ER-targeting therapies, such therapeutic individualization will need to become the norm.

REFERENCES

1. Weidner N, Semple JP, Welch WR, Folkman J. Tumor angiogenesis and metastasis – correlation in invasive breast carcinoma. *N Engl J Med* 1991; 324:1–8.
2. Sledge GW Jr, Miller KD. Angiogenesis and antiangiogenic therapy. *Curr Probl Cancer* 2002; 26:1–60.
3. Engels K, Fox SB, Whitehouse RM, Gatter KC, Harris AL. Distinct angiogenic patterns are associated with high-grade in situ carcinomas of the breast. *J Pathol* 1997; 181:207–212.
4. Guidi AJ, Schnitt SJ, Fischer L *et al.* Vascular permeability factor (vascular endothelial growth factor) expression and angiogenesis in patients with ductal carcinoma in situ of the breast. *Cancer* 1997; 80:1945–1953.
5. Pegram MD, Reese DM. Combined biological therapy of breast cancer using monoclonal antibodies directed against HER2/neu protein and vascular endothelial growth factor. *Semin Oncol* 2002; 29: 29–37.
6. Linderholm BK, Hellborg H, Johansson U *et al.* Significantly higher levels of vascular endothelial growth factor (VEGF) and shorter survival times for patients with primary operable triple-negative breast cancer. *Ann Oncol* 2009; 20:1639–1646.
7. Itzumi Y, Xu L, di Tomaso E, Fukumura D, Jain RK. Tumour biology: herceptin acts as an anti-angiogenic cocktail. *Nature* 2002; 416:279–280.
8. Relf M, LeJeune S, Scott PA *et al.* Expression of the angiogenic factors vascular endothelial cell growth factor, acidic and basic fibroblast growth factor, tumor growth factor beta-1, platelet-derived endothelial cell growth factor, placenta growth factor, and pleiotrophin in human primary breast cancer and its relation to angiogenesis. *Cancer Res* 1997; 57:963–969.
9. Mancuso MR, Davis R, Norberg SM *et al.* Rapid vascular regrowth in tumors after reversal of VEGF inhibition. *J Clin Invest* 2006; 116:2610–2621.
10. Ebos JM, Lee CR, Christensen JG, Mutsaers AJ, Kerbel RS. Multiple circulating proangiogenic factors induced by sunitinib malate are tumor-independent and correlate with antitumor efficacy. *Proc Natl Acad Sci USA* 2007; 104:17069–17074.
11. Ebos JM, Lee CR, Kerbel RS. Tumor and host-mediated pathways of resistance and disease progression in response to antiangiogenic therapy. *Clin Cancer Res* 2009; 15:5020–5025.
12. Cobleigh MA, Langmuir VK, Sledge GW *et al.* A Phase I/II dose-escalation trial for bevacizumab in previously treated metastatic breast cancer. *Semin Oncol* 2003; 30(5 suppl 16):117–124.
13. Miller KD, Chap LI, Holmes FA *et al.* Randomized phase III trial of capecitabine compared with bevacizumab plus capecitabine in patients with previously treated metastatic breast cancer. *J Clin Oncol* 2005; 23:792–799.
14. Brufsky AM, Hurvitz S, Perez E, Swamy R *et al.* RIBBON-2: a randomized, double-blind, placebo-controlled, phase III trial evaluating the efficacy and safety of bevacizumab in combination with chemotherapy for second-line treatment of human epidermal growth factor receptor 2-negative metastatic breast cancer. *J Clin Oncol* 2011; 29:4286–4293.
15. Miles DW, Chan A, Dirix LY *et al.* Phase III study of bevacizumab plus docetaxel compared with placebo plus docetaxel for the first-line treatment of human epidermal growth factor receptor 2-negative metastatic breast cancer. *J Clin Oncol* 2010; 28:3239–3247.
16. Robert NJ, Diéras V, Glaspy J *et al.* RIBBON-1: randomized, double-blind, placebo-controlled, phase III trial of chemotherapy with or without bevacizumab for first-line treatment of human epidermal growth factor receptor 2-negative, locally recurrent or metastatic breast cancer. *J Clin Oncol* 2011; 29:1252–1260.
17. Robert NJ, Saleh MN, Paul D *et al.* Sunitinib plus paclitaxel versus bevacizumab plus paclitaxel for first-line treatment of patients with advanced breast cancer: a phase III, randomized, open-label trial. *Clin Breast Cancer* 2011; 11:82–92.
18. Bergh J, Bondarenko IM, Lichinitser MR *et al.* First-line treatment of advanced breast cancer with sunitinib in combination with docetaxel versus docetaxel alone: results of a prospective, randomized phase III study. *J Clin Oncol* 2012; 30:921–929.
19. Barrios CH, Liu MC, Lee SC *et al.* Phase III randomized trial of sunitinib versus capecitabine in patients with previously treated HER2-negative advanced breast cancer. *Breast Cancer Res Treat* 2010; 121:121–131.

20. Martin M, Loibl S, von Minckwitz G *et al.* Phase III trial evaluating the addition of bevacizumab to endocrine therapy as first-line treatment for advanced breast cancer – First results of the LEA study. *Cancer Res* 2012; 72(suppl.): S1–S6.
21. Broglio KR, Berry DA. Detecting an overall survival benefit that is derived from progression-free survival. *J Natl Cancer Inst* 2009; 101:1642–1649.
22. Conley SJ, Gheordunescu E, Kakarala P *et al.* Antiangiogenic agents increase breast cancer stem cells via the generation of tumor hypoxia. *Proc Natl Acad Sci USA*, 2012; 109:2784–2789.
23. Pegram MD, Pietras R, Bajamonde A *et al.* Targeted therapy: wave of the future. *J Clin Oncol* 2005; 23:1776–1781.
24. Schneider BP, Sledge GW Jr. Anti-vascular endothelial growth factor therapy for breast cancer: can we pick the winners? *J Clin Oncol* 2011; 29:2444–2447.
25. Schneider BP, Wang M, Radovich M *et al.*; ECOG 2100. Association of vascular endothelial growth factor and vascular endothelial growth factor receptor-2 genetic polymorphisms with outcome in a trial of paclitaxel compared with paclitaxel plus bevacizumab in advanced breast cancer: ECOG 2100. *J Clin Oncol* 2008; 26:4672–4678.
26. von Minckwitz G, Eidtmann H, Rezai M *et al.*; German Breast Group; Arbeitsgemeinschaft Gynäkologische Onkologie–Breast Study Groups. Neoadjuvant chemotherapy and bevacizumab for HER2-negative breast cancer. *N Engl J Med* 2012; 366:299–309.
27. Bear HD, Tang G, Rastogi P *et al.* Bevacizumab added to neoadjuvant chemotherapy for breast cancer. *N Engl J Med* 2012; 366:310–320.
28. Ebos JM, Lee CR, Cruz-Munoz W *et al.* Accelerated metastasis after short-term treatment with a potent inhibitor of tumor angiogenesis. *Cancer Cell* 2009; 15:232–239.
29. Schneider BP, Sledge GW Jr. Anti-VEGF therapy as adjuvant therapy: clouds on the horizon? *Breast Cancer Res* 2009; 11:303.

Index